Lecture Notes in Medical Informatics

Edited by D. A. B. Lindberg and P. L. Reichertz

2

Donald Fenna
Sixten Abrahamsson
Sven Olof Lööw
Hans Peterson

The Stockholm County Medical Information System

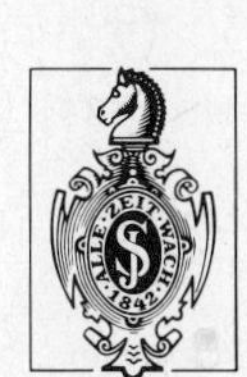

Springer-Verlag
Berlin Heidelberg New York 1978

Authors

Donald Fenna
10–102 Clinical Sciences Building
University of Alberta
Edmonton T6G 2G3/Canada

Sixten Abrahamsson
Department of Structural
Chemistry
Faculty of Medicine
University of Göteborg
Medicinaregatan 9
40033 Göteborg/Sweden

Sven Olof Lööw
Stockholms Läns Landsting
ADB-avdelningen Fack
17207 Sundbyberg/Sweden

Hans Peterson
Stockholms Läns Landsting
Hälso- och Sjukvårdsnämnden
Fack
10270 Stockholm 9/Sweden

ISBN 3-540-08950-0 Springer-Verlag Berlin Heidelberg New York
ISBN 0-387-08950-0 Springer-Verlag New York Heidelberg Berlin

Printed in Germany

Printing and binding: Beltz Offsetdruck, Hemsbach/Bergstr.
2141/3140-543210

PREFACE

The writing of this text arose through the opportunity of one author (D.F.) to spend a sabbatical leave studying the developments within the Stockholm County health operations. The computerization project that had started virtually 10 years previously, focussed on the Danderyd hospital, had received continuing attention in the world scene. It therefore seemed an appropriate site for study for one charged with responsibility for developing computerized hospital information systems.

An intent to assemble a private report became an attempt to write a public monograph when it was discovered that the leaders of the Stockholm project had aspired for some time to put their work more cohesively in the public domain. Since any such publication would be in English and oriented to an international market, the involvement of one extraneous author representative of that market obviously had its appropriateness - in language, interest and detachment.

The resulting book is unusual, if not unique, because of its lengthy and detailed description of one system . Starting from an introduction to Sweden and the local health care system, it proceeds through to detailed descriptions of user procedures, terminal displays, and computer files. Undoubtedly some readers will question the merit in having such detail, particularly as it relates to outmoded equipment and a locally developed programming language. Yet some of those same readers might well be among those many people who ask elsewhere why we should repeatedly "re-invent the wheel" in the computer industry.

One of the obvious reasons why such re-invention occurs is because we generally know so little in the computer industry of what colleagues have created. We may know that another has invented a wheel, but know not whether it is solid, spoked or pneumatic. There is obviously no harm in us inventing better wheels (and few computer applications could legitimately be classed as of the ultimate in development terms). But the development of better wheels requires adequate availability of information on the wheels that already exist.

Our western culture has thrived because of its ability to build further upon its collective achievements. In computer application, however, such accumulating progress has been severely handicapped by the paucity of relevant knowledge. This book is an endeavour toward correcting this problem, modestly in itself and, hopefully, more extensively by its example. The designers of other complex structures have access to a limitless literature on the work of others, touching the elegancies and effeciencies as well as the essential effectiveness of their creations. The information systems practitioner, in contrast, has had little but the basic rules of programming to guide his hand and mind. While one doesn't need an architect to design a dog-kennel or even a small house, one does need trained architects to design good major buildings. The parallel must some day be realized for information systems, and the means provided for the education of such people.

The authors wish to express their gratitude to the numerous people and organizations that have helped, directly or indirectly, the preparation of this document. The Stockholm County Council, the University of Alberta, Health & Welfare Canada and Sperry-Univac have all contributed materially to the project. Rose d'Haene, Sharon Elliott and Heather Bishop have provided the vital keyboard service to convert manuscript into readable text. Many individuals in the health and the computing branches of the County Council suffered silently the probing and questioning that was necessary for the acquisition - virtually always in the English that they use so commendably well but nevertheless must be recognized as their second (or even lesser) language. The text was was prepared and edited via the facilities of the University of Alberta, and the reproducible copy produced by the Government Services Dept., of the Province of Alberta.

In deference to European readers, the comma has been generally avoided as a punctuation for thousands, millions, etc.; the European practice of a space has been adopted. In deference to non-European readers the comma has been abjured as a decimal-place marker; the normal English period has been used.

CHAPTER 1

INTRODUCTION.

Sweden is a land much renowned for its care of its citizens, in health and other matters, and for its advanced technological level. It is therefore not surprising that it should be among the leaders in the application of computers to the medical field. Because of the large governmental involvement in health care it has some advantages in this regard over such countries as the USA. Concomitantly it has some distinctive differences in orientation of its use of computers.

Governmental organization of Sweden.

Sweden is a unitary state with overall responsibilities for health residing with the national parliament - the Riksdag. While responsibility for policy and standards have been retained by the central government, and a major part of health funds passes through the central treasury, responsibility for the provision of health care is divested in the 23 county councils, plus the city councils of Gothenborg and Malmo and the municipal council of Gotland island, which lie outside the county structure. Fig 1-1 provides a map of Sweden and identifies these health authorities, the code letters for the counties being the standard ones used anywhere and everywhere and in themselves indicative of Swedish planning.

With a national population of 8 million people, it is clear that even an average county cannot support a full range of medical facilities. To obviate this problem, seven particular centres - each with a medical school - have been designated to provide a full range of services (e.g including open-heart surgery and kidney transplants) and the country is divided into seven corresponding regions. Fig 1-1 identifies these regions and their centres also. Stockholm, the capital city, is one of the regional centres. Its catchment region is just the County of Stockholm plus the lightly populated Gotland, which has its main connections with Stockholm. With a population of one-and-a-half million, or virtually 20% of the national population, the County alone makes Stockholm the most populous of the seven regions.

Each county is responsible by law for providing all its residents with both outpatient and inpatient care for illness, injury, deformity and childbirth, to the extent that they do not receive care from other sources. Private medical practice exists and the State health insurance authorities reimburse patients for visits to private practitioners, but each county must offer similar services through hospital outpatient facilities or other means, and neighbourhood clinics have a salient and increasing role in this regard.

The County of Stockholm operates 54 hospitals including 13 acute hospitals, plus 28 other inpatient-care facilities. These 82 institutions provide nearly 8 000 general beds, over 6 000 psychiatric beds and more than 11 000 longer term beds. They accommodate about 2 million outpatient visits per year, and the 11 neighborhood clinics, plus mother-and-baby clinics and other non-hospital facilities accommodate a further 1 million. The County employs over 24 000 people in its health-care operations,

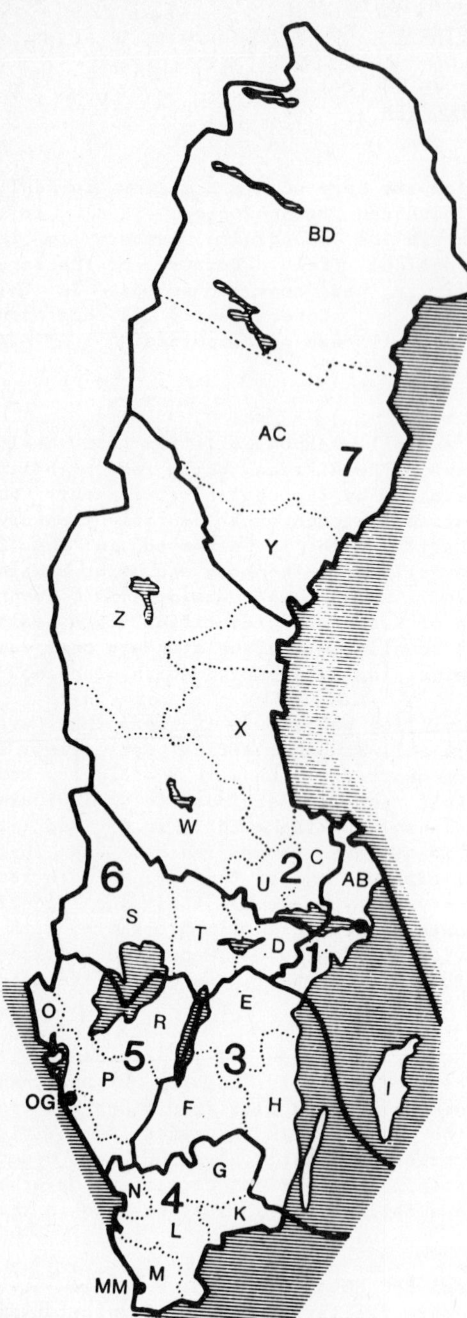

DISTRICTS AND REGIONS FOR HEALTH AND MEDICAL CARE

HEALTH AND MEDICAL CARE DISTRICTS:

County Councils districts:

AB = Stockholm
C = Uppsala
D = Södermanland
E = Östergötland
F = Jönköping
G = Kronoberg
H = Kalmar
K = Blekinge
L = Kristianstad
M = Malmöhus
N = Halland
O = Göteborgs & Bohus
P = Älvsborg
R = Skaraborg
S = Värmland
T = Örebro
U = Västmanland
W = Kopparberg
X = Gävleborg
Y = Västernorrland
Z = Jämtland
AC = Västerbotten
BD = Norrbotten

Municipalities outside the county councils:

I = Gotland
MM = Malmö
OG = Göteborg

POPULATION 1/1 1971 IN THE HEALTH AND MEDICAL CARE REGIONS OF:

1. Stockholm	1 605 596
2. Uppsala	1 247 440
3. Linköping	931 027
4. Lund-Malmö	1 432 731
5. Göteborg	1 446 834
6. Örebro	788 977
7. Umeå	639 177
	8 091 782

FIG 1-1 SWEDEN - COUNTIES AND HEALTH REGIONS

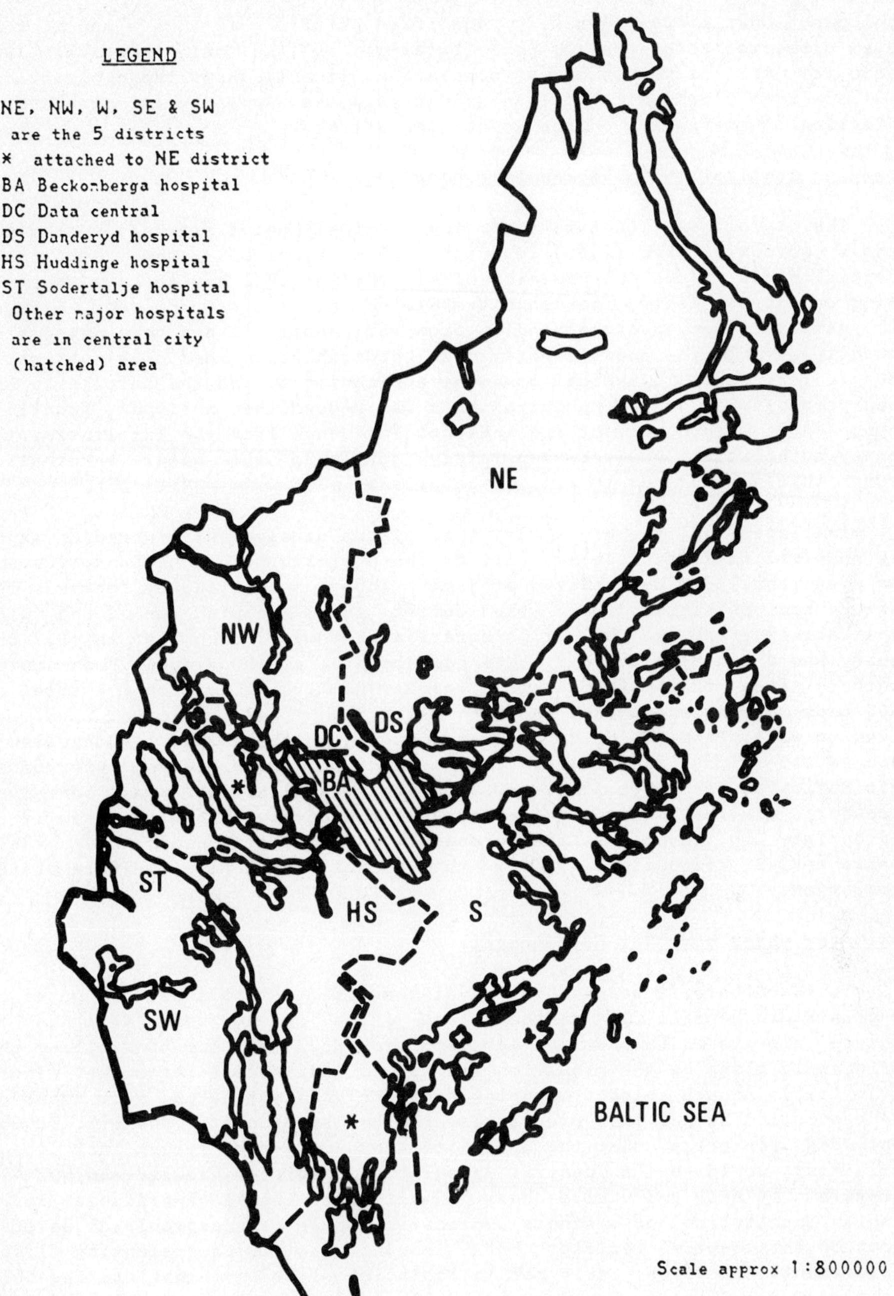
LEGEND
NE, NW, W, SE & SW
are the 5 districts
* attached to NE district
BA Beckomberga hospital
DC Data central
DS Danderyd hospital
HS Huddinge hospital
ST Sodertalje hospital
Other major hospitals
are in central city
(hatched) area
NE
NW
DC
DS
BA
*
ST
HS
S
SW
*
BALTIC SEA
Scale approx 1:800000

FIG 1-2 Stockholm County

including over 1100 medically qualified staff. Fig 1-2, a map of this water-dissected estate, shows the location of the main hospitals and indicates the distribution of population. It also shows the geographical division into 5 districts for management purposes. Appendix A provides a selection of statistics on the County operations.

Computer application in Stockholm's hospitals

The Karolinska Institute - the medical university of Stockholm - enjoys worldwide prestige. Its associated hospital, the Karolinska Hospital, has a special position within the national health care schemes, being one of two central-government-operated hospitals. However, because its patients are overwhelmingly from Stockholm, it has been integrated essentially into the County operations. Leadership in medicine naturally led to leadership in medical computer applications, and the Karolinska has been prominent in many computer aspects far beyond the national frontier. Though not without direct and indirect influence from the Karolinska, the County authorities, however, separately developed the major information system that now spreads to all its hospitals.

Initiated in the mid 1960s, this system development centred on major new hospital facilities being built at the northern suburb of Danderyd, and was even labelled "The Danderyd project". Though so distinctly focused, the system had objectives from the outset that included a County-wide applicability and the fullest integration that was reasonable. In 1962 the County had decided to build a large new hospital at Huddinge - an outer southern area that was changing rapidly from rural to urban. A total of 1600 beds was envisaged and, in tune with the times, consideration was given to widespread use of computer processing in the hospital. Consultants engaged to study the matter recommended an integrated computer-based information system for the new hospital, similar to many conceived elsewhere at that time (1966). However, the County authorities saw it as appropriate to re-orient the proposal, not least because of their comprehensive responsibility for the social and medical welfare of the population.

Basis for major computer development.

To the County it seemed obvious at the time that it should be possible to gain rapid benefit from the computers if a system were designed to include all its welfare activities, and provide a tool for controlling and efficiently planning the provision and use of health care resources. These activities, though highly complex and widely disseminated, must focus on the population rather than programmes or other bureaucratic factors. It was concluded, therefore, that the basis of any computer system for these activities would be a central population register, easily and quickly accessible by many and varied users. Small data banks applicable to a single institution or a single application would be acceptable as an off-shoot of this central register but, though possibly representing local improvements of value, could not in isolation allow anything like the full benefit of computers to be realized in the Swedish context. Maximal benefit was seen as requiring thorough integration. Starting with a central register would allow all types of information and processes be added in a rational and methodical way as requirements and opportunity indicate; starting with isolated applications would require considerable co-ordination and make comprehensive integration difficult. So a cardinal decision was made - the founding of the system on a central population register.

Person identification and population registration.

It is salient to observe at this point something of the Swedish practices in registration of its residents. Every Swedish national and every foreigner granted a residence permit of more than some minimum duration is assigned a permanent indentification number - or 'personnummer'. This number, which embeds the date of birth and some other information, takes the form:

yymmddcrrnc

where

<u>yymmdd</u> is the date of birth (neglecting century) in the sequence year, month, date and using normal numeric notation.

<u>c</u> represents the century being "-" for the 1900s and "+" for the 1800s.

<u>rr</u> is the district of Sweden in which the registration was effected, typically being the district of birth, but for immigrants being a pseudo district - the immigrant office.

<u>n</u> is the sequential number applied to differentiate individuals having the same preceding characters, with even values used for females and odd for males. While this allows for only 5 individuals of each sex to be differentiated it is rarely inadequate. When the number is exceeded - as it could be by homozygous sextuplets for instance - the overflow is accommodated by a reserve region.

<u>c</u> is a check-digit, calculated according to modulo-10 rules.

This 'personnummer' is used very widely for identification in official and non-governmental processes, and is used generally for patient identification purposes. (However, as discussed later, an alternative must be provided, not only for transients in Sweden but because the initial registration takes about two weeks to complete.) The use of 'personnummer' long preceded computers, so is well accepted, though it is not without its skeptics. Beyond this systematic numbering of its residents, and the mere registration of birth, marriages and deaths that is ubiquitous in the world, Sweden operates a thorough system of recording the residents in each locality. This, like the common vital statistics register, is operated mainly by the national church, as agent of the State. Each parish keeps, as a secular function, a record of its residents, and each Swede routinely reports his movements to these record offices. Such diligence on the part of the individual, though eminently in keeping with the ethics of Swedish social democracy, is attributable to more mundane influences; the parish records are the offical records for many purposes; for instance, the address recorded there would be used for social welfare payments. As will be seen below, the permanent address for a patient in the medical information system can be altered only through a communication from the central population registry, to which the parishes report.

Thus, in conceiving the envisaged medical information system as based on a central population register, the authorities had the advantage of a well-established scheme for identifying the population and for recording its changes.

Equipment for the regional information system.

A system that was to be based on the records, albeit basic, of 1.5 million people and yet was to provide real-time access for numerous disseminated uses clearly demanded considerable computing resources in storage, communications and processing terms. However, by 1967 it was possible to see the availability of such equipment, and tenders were invited for equipment of an appropriate specification which, because of the inherent great variation in real-time loading, required that the central processing equipment should have multi-programming capabilities for simultaneous batch and real-time processing.

After tenders were evaluated, the Univac division of Sperry-Rand Corporation was chosen as the supplier, with twin Univac '494' computers as the central equipment. The contract was signed late in 1967 and the initial equipment installed about 6 months later; the full initial configuration of May 1968 is shown in Fig 1-3.

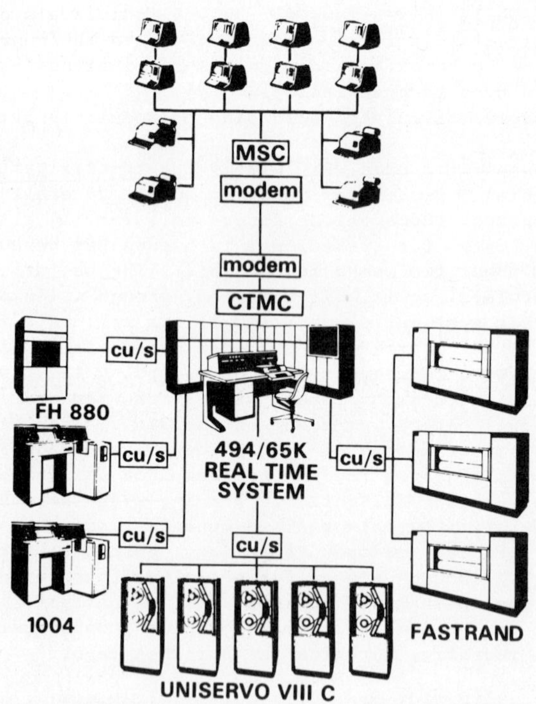

FIG 1-3 COMPUTER CONFIGURATION AT INITIAL IMPLEMENTATION

Basic philosophy of the system

The basic philosophy and main requirements demanded that the system

- cover the whole medical area
- be based on a central population register
- be communications-oriented
- be real-time-oriented
- be functions-oriented

The main aim was to make it possible for the County to follow continuously the morbidity of the total population under its care, and to control the actual utilization of the available resources. The system would also allow, for the first time, a rational basis for the long-term planning of medical care. In these purposes, the system would record all activities related to each patient at the hospitals and other medical institutions, as well as at neighbourhood clinics. The main part of private medical care was also envisaged as being included via the State Insurance Office, and reciprocal advantages, both medical and administrative, to the manually processing insurance office were envisaged from the County's computerization.

Regarding the population register, it was observed that a large amount of data was recorded for a patient each time contact was made with the health-care operations. Name, address and so on were recorded carefully and afresh on many occasions but, what was worse in many regards, the patient was repeatedly asked to recount medical history.

While a restatement of address might indeed be necessary, the recounting of medical history was obviously neither beneficial nor reliable. Often, staff had to request appropriate records from facilities a patient had attended previously. Clearly, in the 1960s even more than today, the inclusion in a computer of the total medical record for so many patients could not be considered. On the other hand, the processing burden of computer, communications and clerk would be reduced if already known information was held by the computer.

A central population register that held both civil records data and pertinent medical information of importance for the care of the individual was the perceived compromise. Accessible to all concerned in the County, such a file would assist overall planning and decrease the need for disseminated records and reference data. Much duplication would be avoided and accuracy would be increased. Security could also be improved.

Clearly the meaningful utilization of such a central population register demanded both the widespread provision of on line terminals and real-time access by the users to the register. Cathode-ray-tube terminals were obviously preferable for many situations because of their rapid display and avoidance of paper output, but a variety of terminals was seen as a need, with low-rate printers being an imperative adjunct at most locations. Real-time access would mean not only ready availability of data for general perusal or use, but would avoid most of the delay in processing that otherwise arises from clerical error. The incoming data could not only be kept minimal in quantity but its quality could be maximal. Many systems that use batch processing, with or without on-line data entry, are able to meet time demands adequately except for the incidence of error entries. However infrequent these are statistically, even one in thousands can entail unacceptability of ensuing reports.

The expression "functions-oriented" in the basic philosophy relates to the manner of construction of the computer-based information system. At the time the philosophy was enunciated there were still people that advocated "total systems", which, in health care, meant the specification, then construction, of a complete system. In Stockholm it was fully recognized that the envisaged system could not be achieved by working out a final package, then developing rapidly the requisite programs and other technical components. Indeed it was seen that not only was the applicational coverage a subject that receded into grey indeterminateness, but that experience would likely cause major revision in some of the distinctly perceived applications. The system had, therefore, to allow easy expansion of its functional domain and easy re-structuring.

Software implications

To meet this last stated objective, the use of a function register was decided upon. Each function, be it patient admission, internally prompted medication notice or whatever, would engage its required programs through the functions register. Should the processes applied to an established function require changes, these could be achieved at the minor level by small program changes but more radically by changing the functions register so as to call different programs. Addition of functions would require extension of the functions register, though not necessarily addition to the program set.

Likewise the programs needed to be detached from the general files, so that changes in files did not compel changes in programs. A general file handling system for storage and retrieval in a real-time environment of the different types of data that constitute the medical record was therefore developed, inclusive of programming languages, compiler, interpretive operating system and various utilities. It was named MIDAS (Medical Information System for Danderyd, Stockholm - and pronounced 'meedas' in Swedish). Under MIDAS, the data stored in direct access memory media is accessed by pseudo-addressing techniques. The records contain data identifiers (or descriptions) that are interpreted by data descriptor registers.

MIDAS also provides various utility programs, particular programs for communications with terminals.

The development effort

As with most projects of comparable size, the 'Danderyd project' was undertaken jointly by the user authority (i.e. the County of Stockholm Health Department in this case) and the main equipment supplier (here the Univac Division of Sperry Rand Corporation, operating through the local Swedish subsidiary). The division of the tasks, however, was rather unusual in that the County had the larger role in developing the special MIDAS software while most Univac programming effort was on the applications areas. For the initial years each of these two parties contributed about a dozen analyst/programmers, with managerial, operator and, later, training staff being additional.

Of 'County' and 'City'

At the time this project started, the jurisdiction of the County of Stockholm was distinct from that of the City of Stockholm. The essence of the latter was the inner urban core, that of the former the surrounding area. However, the County included older communities within very few miles of Stockholm's centre, while the area administered by the City stretched long curling tentacles past these as the City annexed rural land for housing development. The result was two entwined jurisdictions covering one metropolis. Rationalization of Stockholm's local government was overdue.

Rationalization of local government was an important topic of national concern in the 1960s. At the lowest level it produced a reduction of about 75%, to around 700, of the numbers of 'kommuner' - the most local form of government and the one at which, for instance, the responsibility for providing schools rests. For Stockholm it meant a complete consolidation of County-level responsibilities across the extant County and City. Transportation is the other major activity besides health that pertains to County level, and the earlier schism in the metropolitan responsibilities shows in the geography of Stockholm's renowned underground railway system, the 'Tunnelbana'. However, the consolidated authority now operates, through a registered business-enterprize, a highly integrated metropolitan transportation system that pays no respects to old boundaries.

January 1971 saw the consolidation of health responsibility under the enlarged County Council. By that time the initial computer applications had had two years of pilot operation in Danderyd, and the plans for their extension to other hospitals had widened to embrace what had once been the City's hospitals. The computer equipment and associated staff - both operational and programming - not only became concerned with a larger geographical area, but became the general computing centre for the County - 'datacentralen' or, as it is called below in this text, Datacentral. From a beginning in temporary buildings alongside the rising new hospital buildings of Danderyd, this unit now serves its widespread users from its own modern accommodation in an office/industrial highrise in the northern suburb of Hallonbergen.

Organization of the County

The County Council of Stockholm comprises 149 members elected for three-year terms, elections for all levels of government and all localities being held on a common day every third year. The same political parties operate at the county as at the national level, and the Council consequently has 'government' and 'opposition' sides to it.

The full Council meets only intermittently, leaving closer control of County affairs with an Executive Committee of 17 members (plus 10 alternates), appointed by the Council and necessarily reflecting its cross-section. This committee meets once a week, works with the administration of the County's affairs, and is the channel through which all proposals are made to the Council.

Actual running of the affairs, on a day-by-day basis, is the responsibility of full-time paid Commissioners. These are political appointments and invariably filled by the leading politicians in the Council. There are nine Commissioners, six appointed by the government side and meeting as the County Board, and three appointed by the opposition, who function as critical observers. The various operations of the County are assembled into six groups, each the responsibility of a 'government' Commissioner. The six groups are currently:

- Central Administration; Long-Term Planning
- Finance
- Health Care; Buildings & Properties
- Personnel; Education; Culture
- Social Welfare
- Traffic & Transportation

Fig 1-4 illustrates this organization diagrammatically, and shows the main departments, boards and other entities included in each group; as can be seen, there may be several such entities reporting separately to a given Commissioner.

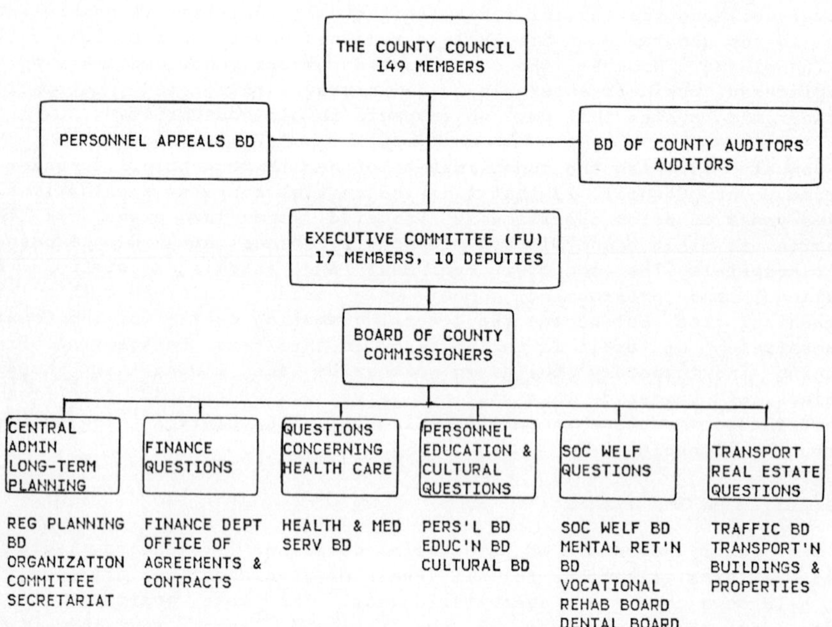

FIG 1-4 HEAD ORGANIZATION OF STOCKHOLM COUNTY

The boards shown under a Commissioner usually include a considerable proportion of political nominees, and oversee in policy terms at least one operating unit, the full-time head of which is non-political. Thus the health and medical care activities are the responsibility of a Director functioning under the Board's direction. The Finance Department, in contrast, has a Director responsible directly to the relevant Commissioner.

Datacentral, including the programmers, is in the E.D.P. branch of the Finance Department, and so responsible to a different Commissioner than is their main customer, the health services. Much of the responsibility for personnel, supplies and accounting within the health operation likewise resides with central units.

With transportation operations detached and under an operating company, health care represents about two thirds of the County employees and a like proportion of revenues and expenditures.

<u>Organization for information systems development</u>

The organizational gap between health staffs and both programmers and computer operations has already been noted. The responsibility for analyzing health care needs and specifying projects, however, rests in the Health and Medical Care Department, namely with the Information Systems Bureau of the Organization and Planning Branch. Here, a small group of specialist staff, after discussions with health staff on the one hand and the computer staff on the other, formulate the proposals for new applications and for further development of existing applications. Since the cost ascribed to health data processing is debited to the Health arm of the County, this group is concerned with the economic as well as functional aspects of developments. It is thus concerned with such questions as use of mini-computers, methods of data input, and just what information to keep on-line.

The organization of the E.D.P. Branch provides three sections under the Manager, these being

- Administrative Section, covering planning as well as general administrative and office service
- System Section, covering design, programming, implementation, maintenance and modification of application systems, plus method development and maintenance of operating systems
- Operations Section, covering operation of the central equipment, technical oversight and support of the remote equipment and communications network, handling of input and output data-media.

Staff numbers in the respective sections are about 15, 40 and 70.

The members of the Systems Section are organized into project teams, each team typically including both 'systems analysts' and 'programmers'. About 15 staff are currently assigned to projects within the medical field, 10 to projects concerned with general administrative systems for the County, and 5 on specifically statistical projects, plus maintenance of the data bank. However, all the staff are assignable to medical or other work as the circumstances dictate, and each new project must compete with all others for these development resources.

It is common practice in the computing field to label the more senior development staff as "analysts", despite the fact that design is at least as important as analysis in their typical responsibilities, and usually more important in the long term than the massive attention to details of pre-computer processing so often encumbered on them. In the case of the

Stockholm medical developments, it must be recognized that most of the analysis is the responsibility of the Health Department, and the senior staff in the project teams at the E.D.P. Branch are even more than usually responsible for design.

Co-ordination of developments

The organizational separation of health and computing add to the more familiar separation of development and user staffs in demanding appropriate co-ordinating machinery relative to deciding both what to do and how to do it. For the Stockholm system there are three committees with overall concern regarding the medical computing.

The E.D.P. sub-committee of the Executive Council, is concerned with all computer developments within the County. The Commissioner responsible for health is a member of this sub-committee, the Commissioner responsible for finance and hence the E.D.P. Branch a conspicuous omission.

The Steering Committee on Medical Data ("Ledmed") comprises the Director of Finance, the head of the E.D.P. Branch and the head of his Systems Section, and an equal number of corresponding staff from the health side: the head of the Organization and Planning Branch, the head of the Information Systems Bureau therein, and one of his project analysts.

The Advisory Committee to that Steering Committee ("Meddata") is essentially medical in character with the head of the Karolinska Institute, the chief medical officers of the two main teaching hospitals, additional members to represent other medical specialties, and a crystallographer from outside Stockholm who, because of his computing knowledge, has been a key consultant from the project's inception.

The Ledmed Committee makes most decisions, using advice from Meddata but within the policy framework and budgetary consequences set by the E.D.P. sub-committee.

Detailed application projects have their own co-ordinating groups as appropriate. Following user or other initiative, any tentative proposal is first evaluated by a member of the Information Systems Bureau, and the raw cost/benefit estimates reported, as a "pre-study", to Ledmed. If the decision favors pursuit of the proposal, a project leader is nominated by the Bureau and an appropriate study group selected from the parties concerned. The resulting "Study Report", specifying the project in considerable detail and providing estimates of more depth than before, is submitted to Ledmed for the decision to proceed or not with development and inplementation. If favor continues, a similar group is formed for continuing co-ordination, with the responsibility for the completed specification, then organization of final testing and implementation testing with the Bureau, and design/programming with the E.D.P. Branch.

CHAPTER 2

SYSTEM OUTLINE - THE APPLICATIONS

Some of the broader characteristics of the System (henceforth the use of this word with a capital letter will indicate the particular system that concerns this book) are already indicated, while the equipment, at least in its initial configuration, has been illustrated. But the philosophy does not define the substance, and equipment configurations invariably change. Before proceeding to discuss in detail the various applications, methods, equipment and techniques, it is advantageous to gain an overview of the System. While this could be given starting from the inside - which would be appropriate for any system founded so determinedly on a central population register - the approach adopted here is to start from the outside. For even with the premise of a central register, the characteristics of the System are primarily influenced by the applications as components of the health care system. What has been included in the central register and what other files have been established is dependent on the applications - actual and foreseen.

REAL-TIME APPLICATIONS

Though many important reports, routine and other, are provided by batch processing, the quintessence of the System lies in the real-time applications. Beyond a few minor enquiry processes, these applications are currently five in total, each generally encompassing many different dialogs through the terminals. The five are

- "Waiting List" covering both inpatient and outpatient needs
- "Inpatient" covering reservation, pre-admission, admission, transfer, discharge, and recording of diagnoses
- "Booking" covering the booking of outpatient appointments
- "Outpatient" covering diagnoses and treatment
- "Chemical Lab" including requisitioning, data acquisition and reporting

Each of these five is effectively a sub-system, and can be implemented for one area, hospital or department without being implemented for another. They are mutually independent, allowing each area or institution to adopt them as circumstances warrant. (Table 13-1 illustrates this, showing the progress of implementation to 1976.)

The Waiting List Sub-system

The waiting list represents the inventory of known, unmet demand, and so one side of the picture to be dealt with in the effort for optimal provision and utilization of services. While the term 'waiting list' is often taken to connote only patients awaiting a hospital bed, in Stockholm it covers outpatients equally, and investigational as much as therapeutic services. Entry of a patient to the waiting list (or additional entry should additional need arise) is initiated by an examining doctor through a "waiting list form". This form passes from the referring doctor to one concerned with the type of demand, who completes the form, identifying the resources needed for the case. Inpatient surgery, for instance, requires at least surgical operating facilities in addition to an available bed, and usually requires certain tests prior to the surgery; these are denoted by comprehensive codes for standard cases and detailed codes for others.

The information in the form is entered into the computer network via a terminal and thereby added to the inventory that is accessible on-line for information retrieval, amendment or cancellation, or automatic transfer to other routines when action is taken to provide the service.

The computer produces, as required, lists of patients awaiting services, by alphabetical, chronological institutional, departmental, specialty, service code, or administrative district order, or in a hierarchy of such orders. Such lists are, of course, prepared selectively for the different users. They are normally printed at Datacentral and distributed by private mail, but can be displayed on terminals immmediately on request, and printed alongside if necessary.

Since the degree of urgency can vary between patients with a given diagnosis, and even more as between patients requiring any given resource, the System has been designed to accommodate some measure of relative priority and expression of absolute time constraint. The (relative) priority code has three values

FF = patient should have service within 6 days
F = patient should have service withing 6 weeks
N = patient can wait more than 6 weeks.

This classification is that of the Social Welfare department, and indicates how the medical services are seen as part of a wider scene. Absolute urgency is represented by entry of the critical date. Segregation by priority and ordering by critical date are naturally available in the preparation of the printed lists.

The waiting list routine was the first to be implemented throughout the County, and, while its reports can be applicable to a segment thereof, the application package is thoroughly integrated across the total area and population. Prior to computerization, very many patients were on the waiting lists of two or more institutions for the one service, so no clear measure of demand was available. With the integration on the computer, such duplication is avoided, and the patient demand rests as a single demand, to be met at the particular facility the County should choose. In practice, each parish has a designated associated hospital (or maybe more than one if some general services are not available at the first). Patients are expected to attend their designated hospital(s) in any emergency, and the County likewise aims to have them assigned there from the waiting list. However, outside of the exceptional procedures available only at the odd hospital, the County offers patients service at non-local hospitals where opportunity exists to serve the patient earlier.

Sixteen terminals spread over 14 hospitals are effectively devoted to the waiting list routine. Besides indirect effect from action in other routines to provide the required service, the waiting list records are also effected by input from the central population registry, notification of deaths and emigration from the County causing deletion automatically of the demands registered for such patients.

Currently the list contains about 31 000 people, and aggregates 36 000 - 40 000 demands.

The Inpatient Sub-system

The inpatient sub-system is concerned primarily with the admission, transfer and discharge of patients to, from and between the various inpatient wards. However, it extends forward of such events to the pre-admission stage, as well as to various post-discharge reporting.

A patient enters the ambit of the inpatient sub-system when, for a waiting patient, an admission date is committed or, otherwise, unscheduled admission occurs. Whichever the moment of entry, the information fed into the sub-system should include intended therapeutic and diagnostic procedures as well as basic personal data and identification of the ward. Estimated length of stay is also required, but can be derived from the above.

For the typical patient, the essential personal data is obtained automatically from the central register of the System, while the statement of intended therapeutic and diagnostic procedures is obtained automatically for the waiting list for most pre-admissions. Thus, for very many cases - in fact a majority of admissions - entry of a patient to the inpatient sub-system comprises little more than identifying the patient, the ward and the date for admission.

Upon admission, the computer proceeds to activate the pre-stated patient procedures. For instance, laboratory tests shown as to be effected upon admission are requisitioned automatically.

Once in hospital, there are special real-time transactions to report the transfer of the patient from one department to another within the hospital e.g. to a technical department such as the intensive care unit, as well as the discharge of a patient, whereby it is also reported to which place he was transferred (home, to another hospital, etc.,). Following discharge the codes for diagnosis, operation (with date) and anaesthesia are noted.

Various patient lists are produced by this sub-system for issue to wards, admission centres, etc.:

- .new patients due the following day (wards);
- .cumulative list of pre-admissions;
- .daily inpatient report (wards);
- .scheduled bed utilization (head physician);
- .detailed list of all inpatients (patients' office, telephone operators and information desk).

In addition there are:

- .bed census reports;
- .monthly utilization statistics;
- .statistics on operations and diagnoses (on request);
- .admission and discharge reports for State Insurance office;
- information for internal and external accounting.

The cumulative list of pre-admitted patients includes all patients that are planned to get a bed in a certain department on a certain day. Even the procedures to be performed after admission are noted in this list. Using this list, it is possible to make alterations to reservations. The admissions desk within the department gets a copy of this list. Every day the different wards get a list "new inpatients tomorrow" containing the patients to be admitted the following day. The necessary preparations for the care of the patient can then be made.

Furthermore, all the wards get a daily list - "inpatient report" - on all admitted patients. Besides the personal data there is information on the expected day of discharge or of transfer to another form of care. Each ward gets two copies of this list. After the physician's round, possible alterations are noted (such as change in expected date of discharge). One copy is then sent back to the terminal where these alterations are registered.

The head physician of the department gets a list "scheduled bed utilization", one for the next three days for each ward separately, and one for the next ten days for the department as a whole.

The patients' office, the information desk and the telephone operators get a list of all the inpatients, in alphabetical order and with information on department and ward.

Through the inpatient routine, bed census reports are produced on inpatients, together with the monthly statistics and, if required, statistics on diagnosis and operations.

By this routine the computer automatically produces admission and discharge reports, which are sent to the State Insurance Office. Information for internal and external billing is also produced.

The Booking Sub-system

The booking sub-system relates both to purely outpatient facilities (including clinics) and to such facilities as x-ray departments, serving both inpatients and outpatients. It is seen as the area of most potential advantage for the application of computers, not only through the better utilization of facilities but also through the indirect effect of avoiding unnecessary delays during inpatient stays.

While aimed at an increased utilization of available resources, the sub-system was also designed with a clear consideration of patients' convenience and preferences. For example, one aim was to facilitate the avoidance of unnecessary waiting time between appointments on a single day. Optimization, in the context of patient and provider terms, rather than maximalization of utilization was the theme.

The sub-system basically keeps records of resources provided and their residual availability, and presents alternative appointments for any stated demand. It deals with the generic service - the 'examination' - which can be investigational or therapeutic, and the particular facility - the 'resource' . Each of these variables is represented by a 4-digit code. The examination identified may be a lung x-ray, an angiogram, a new-patient visit to a medical department, a return-visit to there, and so on. The resource means a particular x-ray machine, a particular examining room, a particular doctor, and so on, that can accommodate, at least normally, one patient at any given time. (Although the term 'examination' in English would normally exclude therapeutic services, and would even be unusual for some diagnostic services, it is used henceforth in this text to mean any of health-care service. The word 'resource' islikewise retained with its wide

Swedish sense.

In seeking a booking, the demand is essentially just for the examination, at least within a specified institution. However, place has been allowed for the demand to be specific as to resource. The situations where resource coding is by doctor provide example of where this is used, in order to have a patient see the same doctor as before, for example. (The coding scheme for resource allows each department or lesser service unit to identify its resources by physical facility or by staff member, but not both ways for any one context. The typical medical clinic sees the resource as the doctor - who may see patients in several different rooms during any one session. An x-ray unit, on the contrary, sees its resources as machines in this regard.)

Operation of the booking sub-system requires entry to the computer of the examinations and the resources, their inter-relationships, the hours of operation of each resource, the duration of time each examination requires, plus textual matter covering both the names corresponding to the codes and explanatory material to be presented to the patient.

The sub-system allows up to nine examinations to be booked in unison, with them divided into two or three groups, if necessary, for explicit attendance on different days, in stated sequence, or even with specific delay between groups. The computer in response always offers, at any instant, three alternative appointments for each examination, and proceeds to further alternatives as required. When acceptable appointments have been established for all required examinations, these are recorded and, if desired, an appropriate notice issued for the patient. This can be printed immediately at the terminal - which is particularly convenient when the booking is being made in the physical presence of the patient - or printed and dispatched at Datacentral. The notice includes not only identification of date, time and service, but also explicit directions to the pertinent reception point and any ancillary directions e.g. no food to be taken in preceding eight hours.

At the close of an initial visit to a clinic, for example, a booking clerk will proceed to make appointments for any tests and other examinations, plus a return visit to the clinic, with the patient in attendance. Not only does this allow the patient to appreciate the alternatives and partake fully in choosing, but it means that the patient knows and has agreed to the consequential appointments before leaving the clinic. A clear notice is in the patient's hand and the clerical work for the clinic completed in this regard - without adding one piece of paper to the clinic's records. The relevant time allowance for test results to become available has been included in the booking. If, at any time, the patient's status needs to be checked or altered, all the bookings are readily visible through the terminal.

Twenty-four hours in advance of each operating day, each reception point receives a printed list of its appointments as known to that point, allowing time for retrieval of files and so on as desired. Late amendments to these reports are available on request via the terminals, as display only or in printed form.

The booking routine is of a nature that allows piecemeal implementation across and even within institutions. Indeed, because of its requirement for documentation of examinations and their times, resources and their hours of operation, and their inter-relationships, it is a routine that necessarily is introduced progressively. Currently it is in use for the orthopaedic and otorhinolaryngology clinics at Danderyd hospital and for the x-ray department and the internal medicine clinic at Huddinge hospital.

The Outpatient Sub-system

With the recording of unmet demand covered by the Waiting list sub-system and the making of appointments by the booking sub-system, the "outpatient sub-system" covers essentially the recording of each outpatient visit. Covering both visits to technical departments and the visits to general and specialist practitioners, the outpatient visits accommodated by the County are multitudinous. The amount of data collected per visit must therefore be severely constrained, and the focus of this application is on the more salient aspects only. Besides the incidence of the visit, any diagnosis or procedures effected are to be recorded, together with an indicator of relative medical status and a note of any use of certain selected drugs.

The general strategy is to make the entry to the computer by terminal, but after rather than during the visit; the doctor continues to make a paper record and a trained assistant makes the entry.

The cumulative record for a patient, in the condensed form indicated, is available from this sub-system for any review of the individual's case. Probably more importantly, the application extends the computer records from the infrequent though complicated inpatient stay to the predominant incidences of health care. It thus brings the potential for a thorough analysis of both the morbidity of the population and delivery of health care.

Unfortunately, even with the restriction to the most salient items, the load produced by the outpatient activities is too great both economically and technically for widespread implementation. The sub-system is, therefore, restricted in its implementation to pilot sites.

The Chemical Laboratory Sub-system

The essence of the chemical laboratory sub-system is the automation of clerical procedures within the laboratory. Both requisitions and results are entered into the computer by laboratory staff, using locally situated terminals. Only results pass within the computer network between laboratory and client department, and no laboratory equipment is connected electrically to the system.

A key intermediate purpose of the sub-system is the preparation of collection lists for the laboratory staff, and of corresponding work lists.

Like the outpatient sub-system, this application for the chemical laboratory has proved too burdensome for general implementation, and is therefore listed for major revision. Such revision is currently underway in the form of the installation of mini-computers within the laboratories. These will bring two conspicuous changes:- a great reduction in the terminal traffic within the central network and progressive on-line connection of the analytical equipment.

BATCH APPLICATIONS

The most crucial batch application is that carried out weekly to update the central files of the System with the changes recorded by census offices. At the output face there are several overnight reports produced on a batch basis within the above sub-systems. However, the most significant batch output is expected to be that analysing incidence of disease, provision of services, etc., for use in planning the health care system of the future.

CHAPTER 3

SYSTEM OUTLINE - THE HARDWARE/SOFTWARE BASE

The selection of Univac '494' computers and the development of the Midas programming software has already been mentioned in Chapter 1. With the growth of the functional and geographical coverage of the System, the original computer configuration has been expanded modestly at the central site, and considerably as regards terminals. The most significant change has been the substitution of more modern disk memories in place of the original Fastrand drums, but no replacement of the two '494' computers is contemplated before 1979. The existing configuration is illustrated in Fig 3-1.

Univac 494 - the central hardware

Though frequently selected for advanced real-time systems involving considerable on-line storage, the Univac '494' is not a very common machine, so a few details of its specification are convenient here. An improved version of the earlier '490', the '494' has a main memory of cores with a complete cycle time of 750 nanoseconds for a 30-bit word. Core capacity is a basic 64 K words, expansible to 262 K; as Figs 1-3 and 3-1 show, Stockholm County has proceeded only to 131K in its expansion. Instruction access is concurrent with the last operand cycle of the preceding instruction, while buffered input/output allowing concurrent i/o transfer and program execution is provided. (Common perhaps now, but not so common in 1962 when the first '490' was delivered.)

Arithmetic operands can be half-word or full-word fixed-point binary, fixed-point binary-coded-decimal or floating binary. No character operations are provided except for input/output of 6-bit alphanumeric characters, allowing 5 characters per 30-bit word. The code used internally is the Fieldata code - the pioneer of code standardization. In single-precision arithmetic, the word comprises a sign plus 29 bits for the argument, 2s-complement arithmetic being used. Storage protection includes one additional bit for parity control per half word, plus upper and lower bounds registers for the executing program.

Input/output transfer is via full-word channels, 12 to 24 of which can be installed in groups of 4. The i/o logic contains a priority control network that determines the order for data transfer requests on the various channels and for responding to system interrupts.

The '490/494' Series was conceived and developed with a clear orientation to real-time applications operating in multi-program and multi-activity modes with background batch programs. Besides the inclusion of the interrupt network, programmable clocks and more general features, this goal required both fast secondary storage and good communications peripherals.

The Fastrand drums installed initially were exceptional in their day for their combination of capacity and access time, with average access time of 92 milliseconds, transfer rates of 31 000 words per second, and capacity per unit in excess of 26 million words. The initial configuration had three such units and virtually unlimited scope for expansion. In addition an 'FH

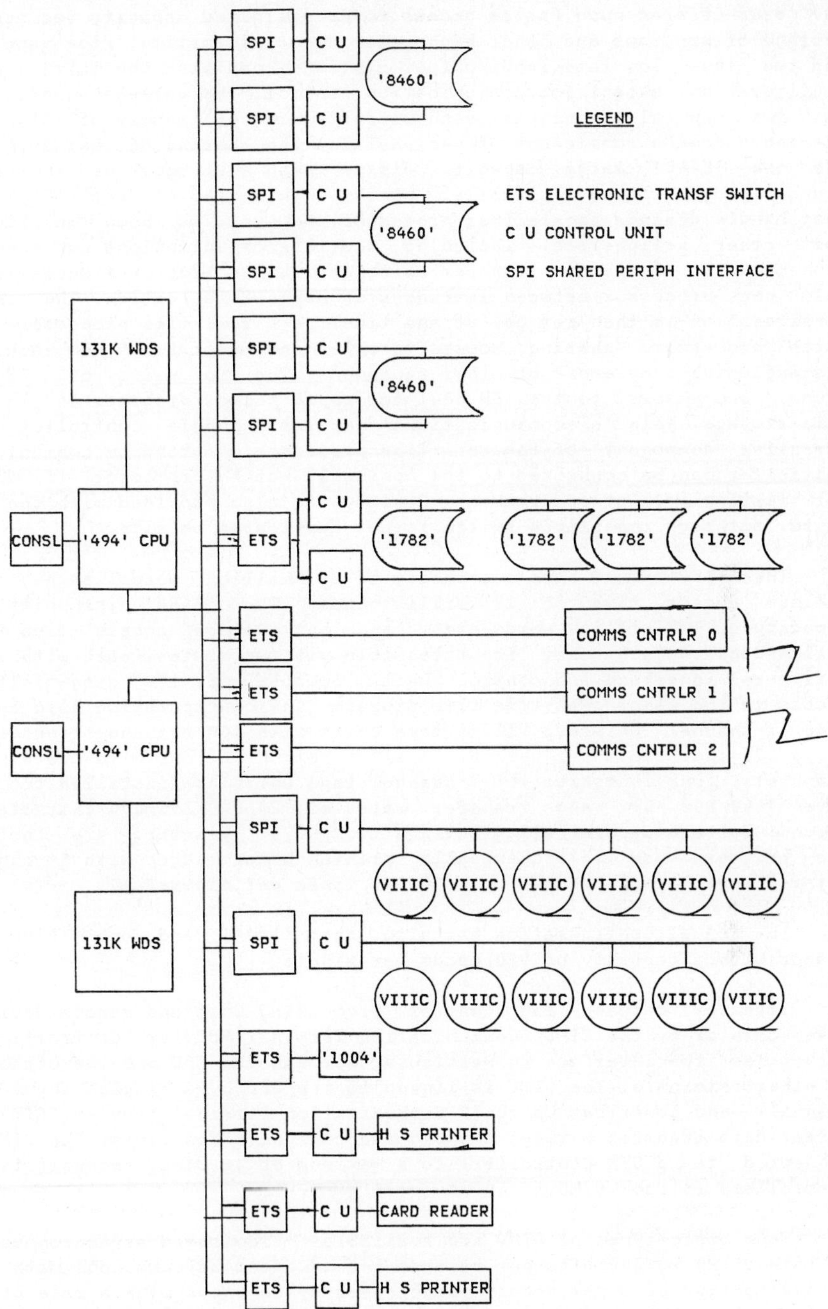

FIG 3-1 CENTRAL COMPUTING CONFIGURATION - 1976

880' drum offered much faster access to more limited capacity for secondary storage of programs and other high-referenced information. Five tape drives and two '1004' low-rate input/output stations completed the initial central configuration, except for communication control. The current configuration has two central processors, each with its own core memory of 131 K words, sharing a common complement of peripherals. The sharing of magnetic tapes and the '8460' large capacity disks, which have succeeded the Fastrand drums, is on a common availability basis, with shared peripheral interfaces that handle demands from either processor. However, as shown in Fig 3-1, most other peripherals, including the telecommunications equipment, are connected via electronic transfer switches, thus making them accessible to only one processor between instances of human intervention. The composite configuration is then set up, at any time, as a real-time processor and a batch processor, sharing access to tapes and major files but each having its exclusive complement of other equipment. The two pairs of 'FH 1782' drums, successors to the 'FH 880' for rapid access programs and reference file storage, join a communications terminal module controller as an essential component of the real-time processor. A stand-by communications controller can be connected to the nominally batch processor if desired, for testing or other reason. Duality is also provided with the '1782' pairs, although the simple switch is not duplicated on site.

The '1782' drums have a capacity of 2.1 million words each, and an average access time of 17 milliseconds. The '8460' disk units have a capacity of 110 million words each, and an average access time of 55 milliseconds. Each unit is accessible via two routes, each with its own peripheral interface and control unit, because of the essentiality of access to the major real-time file storage. The configuration also includes nine 7-channel 'Uniservo VIIIc' tape units with 800 bpi and transfer rates of 96 000 characters per second. To allow communications with certain other computers, four 'Uniservo 16' 9-channel tape units are installed too. They have 1600/800 bpi and transfer rates of 120 000/256 000 characters per second. To take care of all printings two '0770' printers are installed. The printers use interchangeable printband cartridges with 64-character sets. The printing speed is up to 2 000 lines per minute.

The actual configuration has also one '1004' and one '0706' card reader with a capacity of 900 cards per minute.

Transfer between the central processing unit and remote devices is taken care of by the CTMC (Communication Terminal Modular Control), which serves as the interface in particular between the CPU and the cathode-ray or other terminals. The CTMC is linked to the CPU by a single input/output channel, and comprises up to 32 Communication Terminal modules (CTM) which effect data transfer between the CPU and communication lines. The CTMs are connected to a CTM Controller, to a maximum of 16 CTMs, necessitating two controllers in each CTMC.

Four basic types of CTMs are available: - low speed asynchronous with a rate of 20 to 300 bits per second; medium speed asynchronous with a rate of 300 to 1600 bits per second; high speed synchronous with a rate of up to 50 000 bits per second; and dial.

The CTMs arrange data in the format required by the CPU or in the format demanded by the circuit with which the terminal is designed to operate. Input data is arranged in bit-parallel character-serial form for submission to the CPU. Output data is formatted according to the requirements of the associated communication circuit. The CTMs are grouped into modules of two input lines and two output lines. The lines may be used in simplex, half-duplex or full-duplex mode.

Control of the terminal traffic and hence of the contact with the end users (terminal operators) is effected by a group of Communications Supervisors. A special program package was also developed by which operators can follow by display screen the traffic going on per line, and can, for instance, send messages to all terminals or a selected group of terminals about disturbances and so on. The supervisors also accumulate statistical data regarding traffic, errors, availability and so on. A contact person in each hospital is responsible for reporting errors to Datacentral and distributing messages from Datacentral to all operaters.

The Operating System

The operating system in use is 'Omega', level 6, version U. The operating system has to fulfil the demands from real-time and batch-programs in the following areas:

- control programs in a multi-programming environment
- control input/output streams and devices
- allocate core automatically
- allocate appropriate facilities as core, direct access memories, tape between user programs and software utilities
- analyze interrupts and handle error detections and corrections
- co-ordinate usage of input/output channels between programs.

Omega provides a comprehensive library of integrated programs comprising a flexible and powerful executive control system plus a collection of programming language processors, utility routines, and application packages. Through a versatile and effective control language, the executive routine organizes and directs basic computer operations and system activities with the aim of optimizing utilization of computer facilities and system economy. In essence, it is comparable with most other operating systems of its time. However, being operable only on outmoded equipment, it lacks many of the features introduced into operating systems in recent years. Thus there is no 'virtual memory' facility, and time sharing facilities are primitive. However, except for this latter aspect, Omega adequately meets the requirements of the System; in particular, it allows predominant emphasis on servicing real-time demands while providing good background batch service within this constraint.

A catalog of random-access files, the Master File Directory (MFD), is maintained by the system for files which transcend a particular job. The MFD facilitates automatic operation and provides permanent file storage to a collection of individual and independent users.

System integrity is effected through hardware memory-lock-out, guard mode, and software validation of service requests. An errant program cannot destroy the system or other programs in the multiprogram environment. Random access files are protected through the use of file codes and logical file addressing. Comprehensive contingency procedures facilitate recovery from error conditions.

Omega has been in operation many years now and has therefore good stability and safety. On the other hand such parts as sort utilities, conversion aids, logging and accounting are rather poor compared to those of modern operating systems, and the '494' is too old for other than very small changes to be warranted in Omega. Only absolutely necessary correction and cheap enhancements are incorporated.

The Software Package MIDAS

To meet the needs of its transaction-processing real-time system, Stockholm County developed the large software package called MIDAS (Medical Information System for Danderyd, Stockholm). This consists of processes for transaction control and file handling, plus a problem-oriented programming language together with necessary compiler and interpretive operating programs.

The first version of MIDAS was developed in 1968. At that time it was relatively common for large installations to develop their own software packages, but the contemporary lack of any viable software providing for such needs as re-entrant programs, extensive common file handling, and space-economizing interpretive execution - all for the size of operation envisaged - was the crucial factor. The main goal for MIDAS was to develop a flexible software package capable of handling a high volume of real-time transactions exploiting hardware capabilities and using a minimum of core.

A second version of MIDAS was implemented in 1972, the most significant enhancement being a capability to handle parallel transactions. The number of parallel transactions is a system parameter which can be changed depending on the total load of transactions. Currently this parameter is set as high as six during peak hours. In that version, called MIDAS 1.5, changes in the batch aspects were also included. In 1974 and 1975 more enhancements were introduced in MIDAS, for example a new security system (described in Chapter 12), improvement of updating functions, changes in recovery and restart functions, and programs for capacity analysis. The MIDAS software package consists of the following parts:

- programming language
- compiler
- data descriptions language
- transaction control system
- file handling system
- batch system
- utilities

One of the main objectives of MIDAS was to provide all these parts using a minimum of core. While the 131 000-word core of the real-time machine is used entirely for real-time applications during office-hours, in evenings it is used for batch processing in parallel with real-time applications and in night-hours for multiple batch-processing. Fig 3-2 shows the core layout during dedicated real-time running. MIDAS requires also about 50 K words on the '8460' disk and 150 K on the '1782' drums for program modules, file descriptions and working areas.

Transaction control

The main functions of the transaction control system are message handling, security control, and logging of transactions for recovery purpose. In order to protect the medical files from unauthorized use there

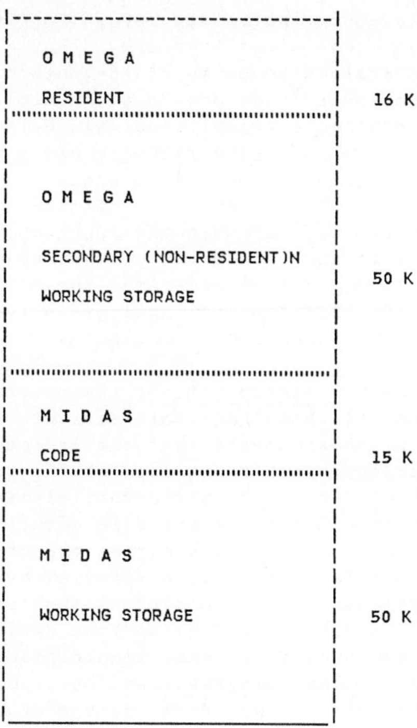

FIG 3-2 CORE LAYOUT FOR THE REAL-TIME ENVIRONMENT

are different kinds and levels of security control. These are described in Chapter 12.

The recovery and restart functions included in MIDAS are based on logging on magnetic tape of transactions and of file updates. The functions use after-looks.

A typical transaction will be described in the following text. The successive allocation of core during the transaction is indicated in Fig 3-3. The only information for a particular terminal which is continually stored in the core is a 4-word terminal reference block. When any activity is started at the terminal the time is recorded in this terminal reference block and a terminal status block is created in core for the duration of the activity. This status block is coupled to various other control blocks and buffers, such as input/output message buffers, then its space is released to a free core chain upon completion. Another core chain connects the released programs and file descriptions, these being kept in core for a parametically defined time to avoid unneccesary accesses.

Unused programs and file descriptions are continually moved upwards in core in order to have as much free core as possible in one piece. Of course, when a free core chain is exhausted these unused descriptions will be discarded to provide assignable space. Another feature in core handling is the core expansion, through rollout of concurrent batch programs by Omega when the available MIDAS core is not sufficient; every 60 seconds the expanded core is reviewed for potential return to Omega for other usage.

A transaction is started by entry of the mnemonic code for the desired function, plus any necessary argument, e.g. KRM followed by a personnummer is used for the retrieval of critical medical data for a patient. The function program which generates the response has a program reference block of two words which is core resident. This block is actually located by use of a name reference block which simply translates the mnemonic function code into a program number. Thus when the function code KRM is transmitted a program status block is formed and the corresponding function program is read into core. The program that generates the screen of critical medical patient data is then executed in an interpretative mode in the MIDAS system.

File descriptions are stored outside the program as will be described in the next section on file handling. Data elements are identified by use of symbolic names ("variable names") that are defined in file descriptions. The variable is described by an identifier of the buffer where the element is stored and by a name identifying the actual element. Only a reference block consisting of two words for the file description is core resident. When a file description is needed at program execution the corresponding file description is taken into core and for every actual record a record status block is generated. The record status block is among other things used for protection against writing, so that during a file update from a terminal no one else can handle the same record. Before the statement using a particular variable in the program can be executed, space must be allocated for the corresponding data by use of an OPEN statement. This instruction requires the name of the file according to the file description, the buffer identifier, and the position of the record within this buffer.

The status blocks (for terminals and programs) have a fixed length of 130 words whereas the file descriptions and programs have a variable length, all dynamically allocated in the working area of MIDAS.

File handling

The data base in a regional hospital information system is by necessity quite extensive. It contains several files stored on different types of memory media and it must allow for wide variations in data structure. A further complication is that major file changes must be possible during the long period of overlapping development and production of the system. The data base control system of MIDAS was implemented in order to fulfil these requirements. As a result, files for direct access with fixed or variable sub-records linked to main records can be created by macro-instruction. Also, by use of file description tables, that define the data structure and file content, and which lie outside the function programs, the programs are independent of file changes.

All the variables, except for 15 internal integer variables, that are used in a MIDAS program must be declared in a corresponding file description. When a particular variable is used the corresponding file description is decoded. A file description defines to the system how the actual data should be accessed, i.e., the type of record and the position within the record. It consists of a master part, describing the file type, and a record description for definition of the file content. The following

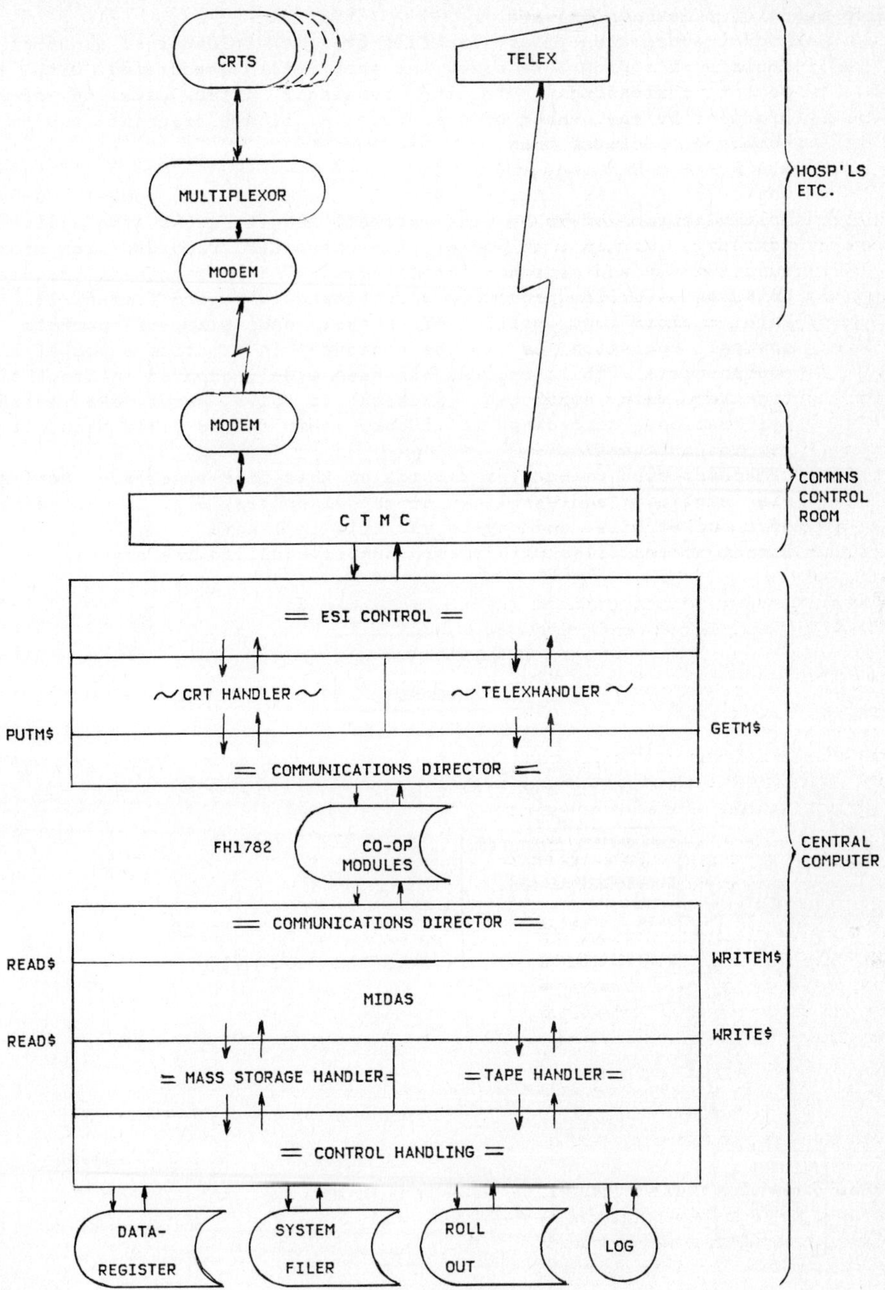

<u>FIG</u> 3-3 SOFTWARE PROCEDURES FOR CONNECTING OF TERMINALS

= INDICATES STANDARD OMEGA

~ INDICATES LOCALLY DEVELOPED OMEGA

three types of files can be used.

- Pocket-addressed files. The file area is divided into a number of pockets of appropriate size, and each record associated with the pocket corresponding to the remainder after division of its argument by the number of pockets. I.e. if A = argument and N = number of pockets, then

  A/N = I + R/N

  where I = some integer and R (0cRcN-1) is pocket number. Multiplication of R by the pocket length gives the relative address. Within a pocket the separate records are stored successively and searched for likewise. This arrangement requires both an overflow provision and a standard record format. It also entails close consideration of number and size of pockets if optimal operation is to be achieved. In practise a pocket-size commensurate with 12 records has been widely adopted in Stockholm, together with sufficient pockets to give about 80% average utilization; according to theory this should yield about 4% of records in overflow.
- Link-addressed files. The records of this file type are accessed via explicit address links stored elsewhere, e.g. in the records of a pocket file, and may be variable in length.
- Direct access files with record number equal to the argument.

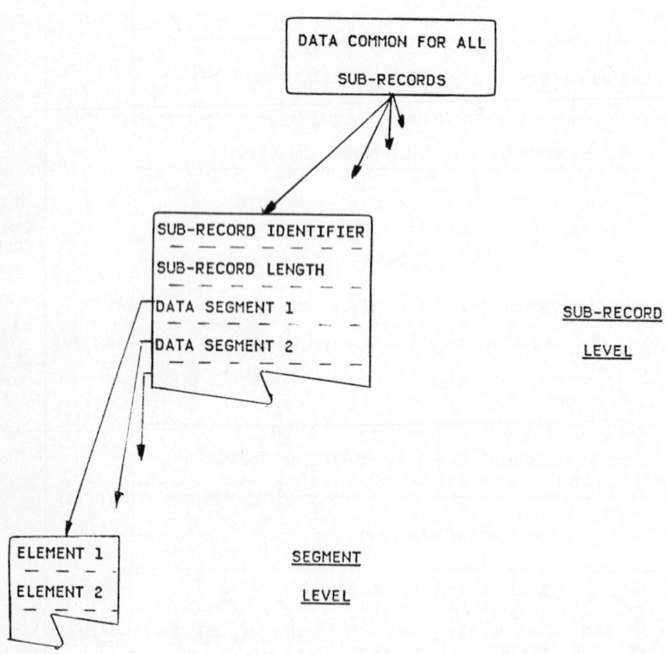

FIG 3-4 THE HIERARCHICAL DIVISION OF DATA

The data structure in each record is defined by a record description. The data content in a record is grouped in a hierachy of three levels. The record can consist of up to six sub-record types. Each sub-record can contain a maximum of six segment types, in which the elements are found. An illustration of the data structure is given in Fig 3-4. For every sub-record an identifier and the sub-record length is first specified, and then follows name references so that a particular element defined by its name in a function program can be identified. The representation of the elements and their length in bits or characters is also defined. The elements can be represented in binary form or in Fieldata character code - denoted by 'B' and 'C' respectively. (The additional prefix 'X' to either indicates an unused field.)

Programming language

A compiler for an interpretive problem-oriented programming language was implemented within the MIDAS system in order to simplify the programming of on-line applications. The language is quite similar to Fortran. It contains the same type of arithmetic statements, logical expressions, jump instructions, and functions for transfer of control between the main program and subroutines. There are in addition special instructions for data transfers between the core and peripheral units, including terminals. Examples of such statements are SEND and RECEIVE, referring to the messages handled in the user programs. There are special functions for bit- and character-handling, for CRT-cursor control, for validity test of variables (e.g., diagnosis codes) as well as combinations of variables, for table look-up in code/text files, and so on.

It should also be mentioned that the MIDAS programming language has been extended to batch processing, as there are usually batch functions such as statistical reports that have to use the same files as the real-time applications.

Terminal network

Currently the system supports over 200 terminals via 38 leased and dialled line connections of speech grade, plus unlimited Telex terminals via 6 lines connected to the switched telegraph network. Initially the network comprised mostly Univac Uniscope visual display terminals. Subsequently the Alfascope display terminal produced by the Swedish company Stansaab has been substituted for most new installations. Associated character printers are either N.C.R. or G.E. Terminal equipment. Table 3-1 itemises for each line the line type and the particular terminals supported.

Performance

Tables 3-2 and 3-3 give monthly statistics on system performance over the years 1974 and 1975. The percentage up-time of the central hardware has been less than many would expect, having been as low as 87.3% in April 1975, and often below 98%. Much of this loss relates to troubles with disk drives which, like the rest of the hardware, are inherently below modern standards in performance. Table 3-3 shows that within the constraints of the performance of the central computing equipment, the availability of the extended network to users has rarely dropped below 98.3.

LINE I.D.	LINE TYPE	LINE RATE	DISTAL END	TERMINALS TYPE	TERMINALS CRT'S	TERMINALS PRINTERS
1.	L	4800	SODERSJUKHUSET	A	15	3 NCR
2.	L	4800	DANDERYD SJH	U	12	2 NCR
3.	L	4800	DANDERYD SJH	U	11	3 NCR
4.	L	4800	DANDERYD SJH	U	10	1 NCR
5.	L	4800	S:T GORANS SJH	A	16	2 TE
6.	X	1200				
7.	X	1200	LIDINGO, TABY, ROSLAGSTULL, LANGBRO SJH, (MULTIDROP)	U	6	4 NCR
8.	X	1200	HANINGE KMN	U	1	
9.	X	1200	SOLNA KMN	U	1	1 U
10.	X	1200	GOVT INSURANCE	U	2	
11.	X	1200	HALLUNDA DISTRICT DOCTOR, SODERBY SJH, HEALTH DEPT. HEAD OFFICE,	U	4	1 NCR
12.	X	2400	NACKA SJH	U	1	
13.	J	2400	EDP-DEPARTMENT	U	1	
14.	J	2400	EDP-DEPARTMENT	U	1	1 NCR
15.	J	2400	EDP-DEPARTMENT	A	3	1 NCR
16.	J	2400	EDP-DEPARTMENT	U	1	
17.	L	50	EDP-DEPARTMENT	U	1	
18 TO 22.	Y	50	MUNICIPALITIES			25
23.	X	1200	SERAFIMER SJH	U	4	
24.	L	4800	KAROLINSKA SJH	A	4	1 TE
25.	L	4800	HOUSING AGENCY	U	9	4 U
26.	L	4800	ST ERIK SJH	U	14	4 TE
27.	L	4800	SABBATSBERG SJH	U	9	5 TE
28.	X	1200	UNIVAC	TESTLINE		
29.	X	1200	LOWENSTROMSKA SJH	U	3	2 NCK
30.	X	1200	HOUSING AGENCY	A	4	4 TE
31.	L	2400	BECKOMBERGA SJH	U	3	1 NCR
32.	X	1200	STATE POLICE	U	1	
33.	X	1200	STATE POLICE	U	1	
34.	L	2400	SODERTALJE SJH	A	5	2 TE+1 NCR
35.	L	4800	HUDDINGE SJH	A	17	7 NCR+1 TE
36.	L	4800	HUDDINGE SJH	A	2	1 TE
37.	L	4800	HUDDINGE SJH	U	15	8 NCR
38.	L	4800	HUDDINGE SJH	U	12	6 NCR
39.	L	4800	HUDDINGE SJH	U	15	8 NCR
40.	L	4800	HUDDINGE SJH	U	14	4 NCR
41.	L	4800	HUDDINGE SJH	A	12	3 NCR+2 TE
42.	L	4800	HUDDINGE SJH	A	20	8 NCR+1 TE
43.	L	4800	HUDDINGE SJH			MINICOMPUTER VARIAN 620.
44.	X	1200	KAROLINSKA SJH			MINICOMPUTER FOR MEDLINE.

TABLE 3-1 LINE TABLE FOR DATA COMMUNICATION NETWORK

L = LEASED LINE　　TE = TERMINET 3000
J = JOINT LINE (INTERNAL)　　U = UNISCOPE 100
X = PUBLIC LINE　　A = ALFASCOPE
Y = PUBLIC TELEX LINE AND TELEPHONE
SJH = SJUKHUS (I.E. HOSPITAL)
KMN = KOMMUN (I.E. MUNICIPALITY)

MONTH	1975	1974
JANUARY	98.6	99.3
FEBRUARY	98.6	97.3
MARCH	98.4	99.1
APRIL	87.3	99.4
MAY	97.9	90.9
JUNE	94.6	96.2
JULY	92.2	94.4
AUGUST	91.0	93.3
SEPTEMBER	97.3	96.0
OCTOBER	99.0	97.0
NOVEMBER	96.2	99.8
DECEMBER	95.3	97.3

TABLE 3-2 UP-TIME FOR THE REAL-TIME SYSTEM (COMPUTERS)

EXPRESSED AS PERCENTAGE OF SCHEDULED ON-LINE OPERATING TIME REMAINING AFTER INTERRUPTIONS DUE TO HARDWARE OR SOFTWARE FAILURES.

MONTH	1975	1974
JANUARY	98.4	98.7
FEBRUARY	98.8	97.7
MARCH	98.3	97.2
APRIL	98.3	96.2
MAY	97.7	98.6
JUNE	98.3	93.9
JULY	98.3	98.8
AUGUST	98.2	98.4
SEPTEMBER	98.6	99.1
OCTOBER	98.4	98.3
NOVEMBER	99.1	90.5
DECEMBER	98.9	99.6

TABLE 3-3 AVAILABILITY FOR CRT-USERS

EXPRESSED AS PERCENTAGE OF SCHEDULED ON-LINE OPERATING TIME REMAINING AFTER INTERRUPTIONS DUE TO HARDWARE, LINE OR SOFTWARE FAILURES THAT CAUSE LOSS OF TERMINAL AVAILABILITY.

CHAPTER 4

THE DATA BASE

The design of a data base for a wide-ranging, expansible, real-time information system demands a compromise between the value of immediate accessibility and the cost of the requisite storage hardware. Because of the myriad details accumulated for a patient, particularly during a stay in hospital, this compromise inevitably results in some dichotomy of the data between continuing and curtailed storage in the real-time facilities, and hence associated off-line files.

Even within the real-time segment of the data-base, the disparity between the histories for different members and progressive expansion to additional functions encourage if not demand some dissection into discrete files. Recent development of 'data base management systems' may obviate such discreteness, except on detailed efficiency terms, but the situation when the Stockholm System evolved was more debilitating.

The typical hospital has medical records ranging, at any one date, from intensively active to veritably archival, covering patients currently in the hospital to patients seen only once and that many years ago. The latter can, of course, become active without warning the following instant; on the other hand the person may be deceased. In designing a real-time computerized information system for such a hospital, it is common to differentiate active (including recently active) from inactive persons, and retain only the barest information, if any, on real-time files for the inactive group. Regional systems that cover several hospitals tend inherently to have a higher proportion of active patients than would the same hospitals separately. The Stockholm System adds to this regional effect by including within its domain the vast majority of visits to doctors as well as to inherently hospital facilities.

The adoption of a central population registry, updated through the State population registries, affects the gross population concerned. On the one hand it adds people as soon as they become residents of the County, some of whom may indeed never avail themselves of the local health care services; on the other it allows withdrawal of deceased persons and also people that have emigrated from the County. While the quantitative effect of seeing the population through the registries' eyes instead of through the hospitals' is hard to ascertain, it must surely be beneficial for a system with such a large outpatient component. The qualitative effect is unquestionable, since it replaces those that have left the area with those potential patients that have moved in. Some pertinent statistics are:-

As of 31 Dec 75

of the 1 497 000 residents
- 740 000 had no medical data recorded
- 530 000 had at least one x-ray recorded
- 475 000 had at least one inpatient stay recorded

<u>During 1975</u>

50 000 people became residents, including
12 000 born in the County's hospitals
52 000 people ceased being residents, including
10 000 through death

In a typical month 18 000 people are admitted to hospital.

Considering that the accumulated records represent only about five years of activity, even for the oldest resident of the County, the above statistics indicate a high level of activity over the recorded population. However, even with today's technology, the retention on-line of all medical data appears economically impossible for such general circumstances. Like so many others, the Stockholm System keeps on-line in this regard a small amount of basic information on everybody and more extensive information on that fragment of the population comprising current patients (the bulk of the latter information passing to off-line archival storage in due course). In terms of on-line files, the dichotomy is achieved by having the H.R. (Swedish 'huvudregister' or main register/file) for the total population and the P.R. ('patientregister' or patient register/file) for the active fragment. Technically, each of these is a complex of files, both functionally and, in the case of the P.R., geographically.

THE H.R. - CENTRAL POPULATION RECORD

H.R. - role

The H.R. is the central data assemblage of the whole System, being that central population register cited as the prime principle of its specification. It provides basic sociological data and acts as the focus for associating the records of the separate medical events in each patient's life.

It is not essential that a person be included in the H.R. to be served by the County's hospitals or by the System. On the other hand, the mere attendance of a person at a hospital, and its consequential processing by the computer of data concerning that person, does not itself result in the person being included in the H.R. Though there are some exceptions, the H.R. is effectively a register of all current residents of the County - updated, weekly in batch mode, by advice from the census office.

Beyond this fundamental role, the H.R. was designed also to provide, by real-time response to enquiries,

- a brief summary of the person's contacts with the health services
- advice of any medical factors that could be critical in the management of the person admitted as an emergency case
- reference to x-rays performed anywhere in the County on any person.

H.R. - general contents

The contents of the H.R. are divided into four groupings viz:-

<u>Census data</u> including

PERSON-NUMB[1] ('personnummer')
name
address - in postal form and geographic code
profession/occupation
nationality
civil status and date of its last change
whether person is of sound mind
identity of spouse or guardian

Previous inpatient care data, being for each case
hospital and department
date and terms of admission
date and terms of discharge
coded diagnoses
coded operations, with anaesthesia codes

Critical medical data
telephone numbers - home and business
blood group
critical diseases (eg. diabetics, haemophilia - see Table 4-1)
drug extrasensitivities
vaccinations - year, month, type.

The first of these groupings covers information that is essential for the person to be included in the H.R., and which is obtained from the census registries; just one corresponding record is required per person, as only current information is needed. This data is referred to as "C.F.U. data".

The second and fourth groupings represent compact summaries of medical events, each grouping necessarily having to have an unlimited number of corresponding records for any patients. Though the State Insurance Office and other sources may provide such data, these records are primarily derived automatically from the detailed applications within the System.

The Critical Medical Data grouping is more heterogeneous, ranging from the socialogical telephone number to the clinical blood group. Though the diseases, sensitivities and vaccinations occur without specific limit, this grouping can be seen as a hospital-amendable adjunct to the census information, with one variable length record per patient. Its contents clearly have various origins rather than being the summary of any one event.

A fifth grouping - general outpatient record - has been conceived but is not included currently because of the very limited coverage of the outpatient sub-system, and hence of the readily available data.

H.R. - strategy

The strategy for the H.R. is to provide a central record, keyed by PERSON-NUMB and containing essentially just the CFU data, with pointers to the medical data. Since the PERSON-NUMB ranges almost randomly over a 9-

◊◊◊◊◊◊◊◊◊◊◊◊◊◊◊◊◊◊◊◊

[1] terms in block print with broken underlining are names of data fields. Where appropriate, examples of their data values are given in Appendix B

CONDITION	WHO DISEASE CODES
DIABETES MELLITUS	26009-26099
HYPOPARATHYROIDISMUS	27110-27119
PORFYRI	28940-28941
DYSGAMMAGLOBULINAEMI	28950
COAGULATION DISEASES	29500-29509
	29600-29619
BLOOD ILLNESSES	29799
	20400-20448
EPILEPSY, SPASMODICAL STATES	35300-35339
	78020
HEART DISEASES	43301,43302
	43307,43308
	43311,Y1900
MYASTHENIA GRAVIS	74400
CORTISONE TREATMENT	--
ANTICOAGULANT TREATMENT	--

TABLE 4-1. ILLNESSES AND TREATMENTS REGARDED AS "CRITICAL".

decimal-digit range, but only about 1 1/2 million values occur in this context, a pocket file was indicated for the CFU data. With the enunciated policy of 12 records per pocket and a nominal occupancy of 80%, about 150 000 pockets would be required.

CFU FILE

CFU RECORD (LENGTH 25 WORDS)

B30	PNR
C36	NAME (SURNAME, FORENAMES)
C27	STREET ADDRESS
C13	POST TOWN
C10	PROFESSION/OCCUPATION
C 2	NATIONALITY
B13	NON-MEDICAL PENSION DATA
B 4	CIVIL STATUS
XB 8	
B 1	1 = NOT OF SOUND MIND
B30	SPOUSE OR GUARDIAN'S PNR
B 7	CENSUS YEAR
B 3	NON-GEOGRAPHIC REGISTRATION (EG. 5 = ROYAL HOUSEHOLD)
B18	CODED ADDRESS FOR COUNTY-MUNICIPALITY-COMMUNITY
B 7	GEOGRAPHIC CENSUS TRACT
B17	PROPERTY NUMBER WITHIN TRACT
XB 8	
B17	POST CODE
XB13	
B30	LINK ADDRESS TO MEDICINE FILE

TABLE 4-2. DATA DESCRIPTION OF CFU FILE OF H.R.

(POCKET FILE : POCKET SIZE = 330 WORDS; 110,311 POCKETS. ONE RECORD PER PERSON.)

H.R. - storage of CFU data

Table 4-2 shows the precise contents of the general CFU record in the H.R., which total 25 words per person. However, it is clear from these listed contents that not only are many fields applicable only to adults, but that much of the balance is common for the separate members of one family. While the latter aspect was not deemed sufficiently potent to warrant a common family record of any form, the two aspects together were seen as justifying the separation of minors and the definition for them of a much reduced head record. This is shown in Table 4-3; it consists essentially of only the personal name of the given PERSON-NUMB, plus the PERSON-NUMB of the guardian and the normal pointer to the medical data. However, a considerable amount of space is reserved for future use, bringing the record to 11 words, but still less than half the adult CFU record.

MINORS CFU FILE

MINORS CFU RECORD (LENGTH 11 WORDS)

B30	PNR
C36	NAME (SURNAME, FORENAMES)
XB24	
B30	GUARDIAN'S PNR
B30	LINK ADDRESS TO MEDICINE FILE

TABLE 4-3. DATA DESCRIPTION OF MINORS CFU FILE OF H.R.

(POCKET FILE; POCKET SIZE = 198 WORDS; 22,229 POCKETS. ONE RECORD PER PERSON.)

The current boundary between 'adult' and 'minor' for the System is the calendar-year-end when the person is 17 years old. With such division, there are about 1 100 000 adults and 400 000 minors. (However, recent sociological trends - for instance, an increased occurrence of children leaving home before this age - are tending to negate the economy of this dichotomy. Consideration is therefore being given to standardizing on the larger format.)

When these two files were originally designed the respective populations were 1 056 853 and 319 865. On the standard criterion of 80% packing with 12 records per full pocket, this indicated about 110 000 pockets of 330 words (10 segments) each for the adult file; the prime 110 311 was adopted. For the minors file, with its distinctively small record, a criterion of 85% packing with 17 records per full pocket was used, leading to the prime 22 229 as divisor and number of pockets. (Strictly these numbers did not need to be fully prime, but there is sufficient irregularity in the distribution of the digits in PERSON-NUMB, even after conversion of month-day to a composite number, to necessitate relative primes of considerable complexity.)

The actual contemporary totals in the respective files are

900 000 persons in the adults pockets
300 000 persons in the minors pockets
giving respective utilities of 73% of the 37 000 000 words and 80% of the 4 400 000 words assigned.

The overflow for adults and minors is in one common CFU overflow file, where, being a linked file, each record occupies a whole 33-word segment. The 179 000 overflowing records thus occupy 6 000 000 words with a utility of 65%. The gross assignment is 7 000 000 words, producing a true utility of only 57%.

H.R. - form of PERSON-NUMB

As can be seen from Table 4-2 & 4-3, the PERSON-NUMB by which the H.R. is keyed is in a 30-bit form - i.e. occupies precisely one computer word. Since the external form includes nine decimal digits plus a century indicator, exclusive of the redundant check digit, some adjustment is required to achieve the placement in one word. This is achieved by conversion of the inefficient identification of month and day from four digits to three, in fact to the values 1-366 being the actual day of the year, and placement of these digits in front of the remaining ones. Placing also the century indicator as the sign bit of the word thus gives a value in the range k366 999 999, or within k2pw. If jjj represents the so-called Julian date number for the day within the year, then the

yymmdd∂rrnc

of the external PERSON-NUMB, described in Chap 1, becomes

∂jjjyyrrnc,

albeit with a recalculated value for c. This altered internal form will also be referred to as PERSON-NUMB or, more abbreviatedly, PNR.

H.R. - storing the medical data

As already observed, the medical data of the H.R. requires both variable-length records and an unlimited number of logical records for any one person. The design of the H.R. provides for all the medical data pertaining to any one patient to be effectively consolidated in disk storage, and accessed via the one link address at the end of the pertinent CFU record.

The relevant file description is shown in Table 4-4, and can be seen as providing a brief lead record plus separate descriptions for x-ray, inpatient and critical medical data purposes. The latter two of these have multiple-occurrence groups, in the one for operations and diagnoses, in the other for critical diseases, critical sensitivities and vaccinations.

Each of these records other than the lead record is distinguished as to type by a code number in its first nine bits, with the next nine bits giving the length of each particular data record (these common fields being defined in a phantom General record). All these records for any one patient are then concatenated behind the pertinent lead record, producing a consolidated medical history that must be searched by type as well as date etc., for any particular data. The link in the CFU record gives the connection to the lead record of this ensemble, which can readily include other types of data as development occurs. The overall concept is illustrated in Fig 4-1.

MEDICAL FILE

```
LEAD RECORD. OCCURS ONCE.
          B 3   NON-ZERO = IN USE
          B12   NUMBER OF RECORDS (MAX )
          B15   NUMBER OF WORDS IN RECORD-ENSEMBLE
          B30   PNR
GENERAL RECORD (COMMON FIELDS) NO OCCURRENCE
          B 9   RECORD TYPE
          B 9   NUMBER OF WORDS IN SUB-RECORD
SV RECORD (INPATIENT STAY)
          B18   SEE GENERAL RECORD (RECORD TYPE = 003)
          B10   INSTN TO WHICH ADMITTED
          B 2
          B17   DATE OF ADMISSION
          B16   DATE OF DISCHARGE
          B 3   ADMISSION CODE (ADMC)
          B 3   DISCHARGE CODE (DISC)
          B 3   ORDINAL OF DIAG THAT CAUSED DEATH
          B 4   NUMBER OF DIAGNOSES (GROUP 2)
          B 4   NUMBER OF OPERATIONS (GROUP 1)
     GROUP 1 (OPERATION) OCCURS 0 -
          B 4   ORDINAL OF DAY OF STAY
          B14   OPERATION CODE (OPNC)
          B10   ANAESTHESIA CODE (ANEC)
         XB 2
     GROUP 2 (DIAGNOSIS) OCCURS 1 -
          C 5   DIAGNOSIS CODE (ICDC)
RTG RECORD (X-RAY)
          B18   SEE GENERAL RECORD (RECORD TYPE = 002)
          B10   INSTN PERFORMING X-RAY
         XB 2
          B17   DATE OF X-RAY
          B10   DEPT PERFORMING X-RAY
         XC 2
          B10   PART OF BODY X-RAYED
          B10   TECHNICAL METHOD (CODE)
          B10   FINDING (CODE)
         XB21
KRM RECORD (CRITICAL MEDICAL DATA) OCCURRENCE 0 OR 1.
          B18   SEE GENERAL RECORD (RECORD TYPE = 001)
         XB12
          B15   TELEPHONE AREA CODE - HOME
          B15   TELEPHONE AREA CODE - WORK
          B30   TELEPHONE NUMBER - HOME
          B30   TELEPHONE NUMBER - WORK
          B 4   BLOOD GROUP (ABO TO RHESUS).
          B 1   1 = RARE BLOOD TYPE
          B 2   NUMBER OF TIMES TYPED (3 = 3 OR MORE)
          B 4   NUMBER OF CRITICAL DISEASES RECORDED
          B 4   NUMBER OF EXTRASENSITIVITIES RECORDED
          B 4   NUMBER OF VACCINATIONS RECORDED
         XB10
     GROUP 1 (CRITICAL DISEASE) OCCURS 0 -
          B 6   DISEASE (CODE)
     GROUP 2 (EXTRASENSITIVITY) OCCURS 0 -
          B 6   TYPE OF EXTRASENSITIVITY (CODE)
     GROUP 3 (VACCINATION) OCCURS 0 -
          B 7   VACCINATION (CODE)
          B 4   MONTH OF VACCINATION
          B 4   YEAR
```

TABLE 4-4. DATA DESCRIPTION OF MEDICAL FILE OF H.R.

(LINKED FILE. NO FIXED LIMIT OF SIZE OF RECORD-ENSEMBLE FOR ANY ONE PERSON.)

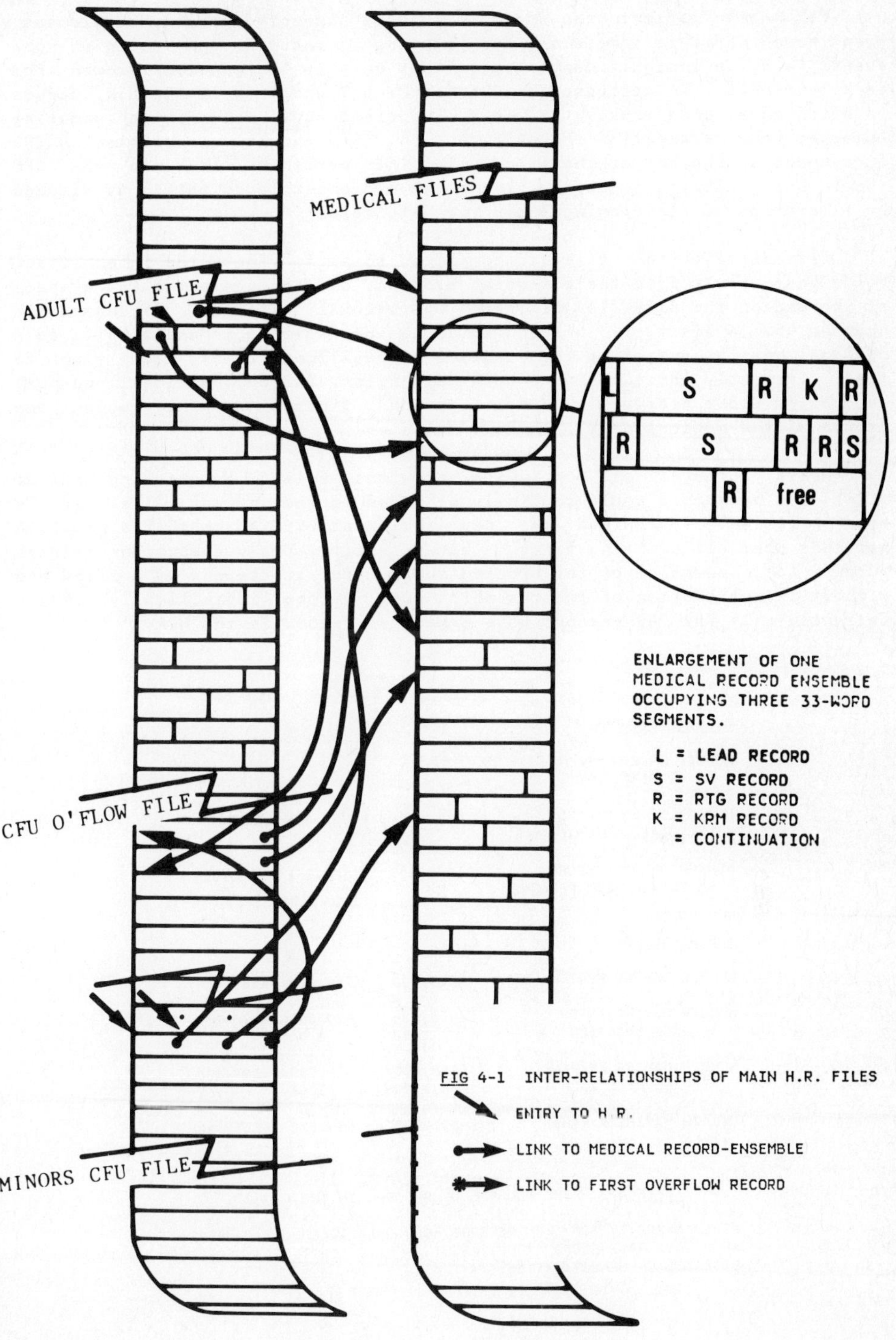

FIG 4-1 INTER-RELATIONSHIPS OF MAIN H.R. FILES

For each patient the ensemble must be augmented as time progresses. Even though there is some scope for removing or reducing the record of some events (e.g. an insignificant x-ray), this entails a general growth for each ensemble. As discussed in Chapter 2, all updating of the H.R. occurs in batch mode, and weekly or less in frequency. Where such updating enlarges any patient's ensemble, the enlarged ensemble is written in the free space at the end of the file, with the pertinent link in the CFU record being altered accordingly, and the old ensemble is marked as disused by alteration of its opening 3-bit field to zero.

Periodically the file is compacted so as to remove the intermittent voids that result from the foregoing process, and aggregate the spare space at the end of the file. To minimize operational problems, discussed in Chapter 5, a limit of 5 million words has been set to a Medical file as a physical entity, entailing the creation of additional files from time to time. Currently there are nine such data files, and an additional one must be created about yearly. Table 4-5 provides figures on the amount and growth of the medical data of H.R.

While turnover of population provides relief in existing Medical files, and newcomers could routinely be added to the newest file, it is more efficient to spread the new increment of space that a new file provides over all existing files. The necessity for compaction relates purely to consumption of the blocked spare space at the end of a file, and without redistribution of records this must become impractically small. Currently only 750 000 persons have a medical record in the H.R.

	JAN 75	JAN 76	CHANGE
OVERALL FIGURES			
NUMBER OF CFU RECORDS (= POPULATION COVERED)			
NUMBER OF SV RECORDS (= TOTAL ADMISSIONS)	766,890	1,002,456	+235,566
NUMBER OF RTG RECORDS (= TOTAL X-RAY REPORTS)	1,070,800	1,879,161	+808,361
THE PATIENTS			
NUMBER HAVING MEDICAL DATA	615,600	750,605	+135,005
NUMBER HAVING AN SV	408,826	479,060	+ 70,234
AVERAGE SVS EACH	1.88	2.09	+ .21
NUMBER HAVING AN RTG	358,407	535,707	+199,300
AVERAGE RTGS EACH	2.99	3.51	.62
NUMBER HAVING A KRM*	552,380	684,222	+131,842

TABLE 4-5. THE NUMBERS OF RECORDS IN THE H.R.

*THE MAJORITY OF KRM RECORDS HOLD ONLY TELEPHONE NUMBERS. ABOUT 40% HAVE BLOOD GROUP, ABOUT 3% HAVE CRITICAL MEDICAL DISEASES OR SENSITIVITIES.

H.R. - Administration and Name files

Besides the files for census data and for medical data, the H.R. complex contains two other files of a service nature. One, the Administration file, comprises 2, 112 words of control data concerning sizes of the associated files and similar matters. The other is the Name file, being a lexicographically ordered list of the personal names in the H.R., each with its PERSON-NUMB. Only the first five characters of the name are held, giving with the PERSON-NUMB just two words per person. This list is provided to allow practicable searching of the H.R. for people known by name but incompletely, at most, regarding PERSON-NUMB. To simplify searching, an index list is added at the front, being effectively a sub-list of every thousandth person.

Since the PERSON-NUMB embeds birthdate and sex, this special file provides for selective searching by these parameters as well as the name component. For any given name part, multiple records are in order of PERSON -NUMB.

THE P.R.s - PATIENT FILES

P.R. - coverage

Whereas the H.R. covers all residents, the P.R.s provide, as we have seen, in-depth detail for that modest fraction of the population currently active as patients. Because these people have an association with a particular institution for the current treatment or investigation, and despite the storage inefficiency that results for patients current with two or more institutions, the recording of this detailed information has been divided into distinct files for distinct institutions. Each file has, of course, the same description and functions identically within the System, so it suffices to discuss one such file, in the context of one institution. [A single P.R. does not have to relate to just one hospital; the System allows it to be a group of hospitals].

P.R. - the RESV-NUMBER

Like the H.R., a P.R. has one central record for each person it covers, plus an unspecified number of associated records. And like the H.R. again, it is keyed on the patient's identification number. However, whereas any person in the H.R. must have the standard Swedish personnummer, such a condition does not apply to the P.R. because of tourists and short-term residents that require health care while in Stockholm. For these exceptions, and such others as residents for whom the standard number cannot be ascertained, a special reserve number is used. Assigned by the computer immediately upon request for any individual, this special number is written in the distinctive form

yyhh-aaaaac

where

yy indicates the current year

hh is the number of the P.R. concerned

aaaaa is a progressive sequence number within the above, separately odd for males and even for females.

c is the modulo-10 check digit.

This entity is referred to as RESV-NUMBER or RNR henceforth; its assignment is discussed in Chapter 5.

Thus distinctive from any PERSON-NUMB when printed in punctuated form, the internal form of RESV-NUMBER is also distinctive internally by manipulating it arithmetically so as to lie between the 367 000 000 that is the maximal internal value for PERSON-NUMB and the 2^{29} that is the maximal value for a single computer word. However, an additional binary indicator is often placed in a record. The exclusion of birthdate from RESV-NUMBER, done to avoid any obstruction in the recording, for instance, of an unconscious and unidentifiable patients, but more generally to avoid reliance on less formal advice, also necessitates the birthdate being recorded separately from the identification number.

It should be noted also that residents of other Swedish counties, and even newly arrived residents of Stockholm County, can require inclusion in the P.R. under their standard numbers although not included in the (current) H.R.

P.R. - strategy

As with the H.R., a P.R. is actually a collection of files, in this case a pocket file of head records plus files corresponding with the different sub-systems in which a patient can be active, e.g. inpatient, outpatient, chemical laboratory. The head record for a patient indicates which sub-systems the patient is currently active within, and cites the hardware link address to the associated record for each.

In designing the P.R., allowance was made for additional sub-systems to those currently developed; one other, for bacteriology, was at one point in use but was later discontinued. The design in current use also bears some imprint from earlier design plans that have been discarded, particularly the one-time plan for inclusion of the waiting list in the P.R. instead of the separate integrated waiting list design described later. Less intentionally in planning terms, the division of data between head record and sub-system records is not ideally organized, the head record, for instance, including several fields pertaining only to inpatient activity.

There are five sub-system files currently in use, namely

VL - a heritage of the waiting-list plan
SV - relating to the inpatient sub-system
DBP - relating to the booking sub-system
OV - relating to the out-patient sub-system
KEM - relating to the chemical laboratory sub-system,

each being a linked file from the head records. The relationship is illustrated in Fig 4-2.

P.R. - the head record

Beyond the identification by number and name of the patient, the head record of the P.R. is largely a 'housekeeping' record concerned with recording the patient's status in this multi-functional file complex. Not only does this cover which of the sub-systems the patient is currently active within, with appropriate link address for each, but, because of the scheme for transferring data from the P.R., data must be kept regarding the completed records awaiting storage, and the repetitions even within the normal P.R.- retention timescale. For instance, it is possible for a patient to have two or even more inpatient stays incomplete awaiting final

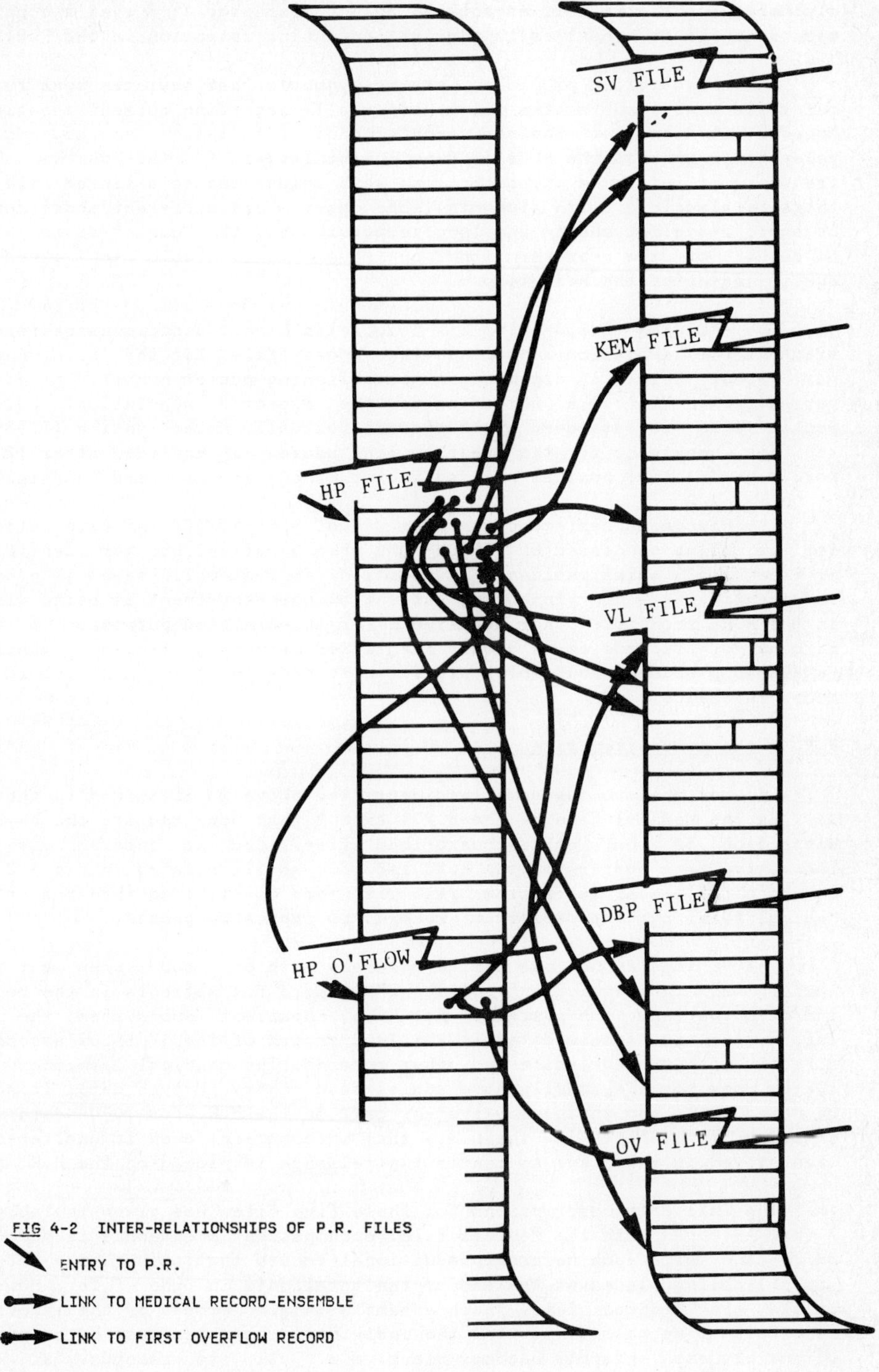

FIG 4-2 INTER-RELATIONSHIPS OF P.R. FILES

discharge reports as well as actual lack of discharge, and even a completed record may be so recent as to require continuing retention in the P.R.

The head record provides a status synopsis that obviates some further reference to the sub-system files, especially regarding current inpatients. However, it does not include such common information as address and telephone numbers, the VL file functioning largely for this purpose. While frequency of reference may merit some such relegation to a linked file, and there is also (e.g. with students) some cases where different addresses may be appropriate for short- and long-term purposes, this use of VL is largely a result of the earlier line of development. Table 4-6 gives the specification of the head record.

The PNR/RNR field plus its associated binary discriminator form the argument for identification within this pocket file, but the main numeric part alone serves as argument for establishing pocket number. The divisor varies from P.R. to P.R. according to the expected population, but the pocket size is standard at 12 records (actually necessitating 13 33-word segments when space for the overflow link address is included after 12 33-word records). The nominal packing factor of 80% is also used uniformly.

The circumstances enunciated for use of RESV-NUMBER indicate potential for it being succeeded by PERSON-NUMB when a patient becomes identifiable or becomes a Swedish resident. In addition, no systematic means is provided for identifying a new-presenting patient at one department as being already in the P.R. from some other department for an unrelated purpose. To allow merging of records for a doubly identified person, particularly where the PERSON-NUMB becomes available, provision is made in the head record for cross-reference.

P.R. - the sub-system files

Each of the sub-system files identified above is organized in the same way as the Medical file of the H.R., except that none require the physical dissection of that earlier-described file, and is entered via the respective link address in the head record - as illustrated in Fig 4-2. The coverage of each sub-system file is more constrained than that of the Medical file, but the variety of records is typically greater.

The VL file is not associated uniquely with one sub-system but acts largely as the equivalent of the CFU record for patients in the booking and/or outpatient sub-systems. For the inpatient sub-system the same information is accommodated in the lead record of the SV file, associated directly with the admission and other records. The chemical laboratory sub-system does not necessarily have address and other CFU-type data. It should be noted that, though the sub-systems call on the H.R. for CFU data when entering a patient in the H.R., that information, even if unaltered, is then stored in the P.R.; no continuing reliance is placed on the H.R.

The full data descriptions for these five files are given in Tables 4-7 thru 4-11. As with the Medical file, each patient's ensemble is added to, on the end, with each necessary additional record that arises, the extended ensemble being placed at the end of the total data in the file. However, unlike the Medical file, each ensemble is also eroded by the removal of records as time passes, so that the individual ensembles must be compacted. Ultimately each ensemble becomes blank, i.e. all its records, at least

HP FILE

```
HEAD RECORD           (RECORD LENGTH 33 WORDS)
              B30   PNR/RNR
              B30   PNR-EQUIVALENT DATE OF BIRTH IF RNR.
              B30   THIRTY BINARY FLAGS CONCERNED WITH
                    STATUS OF PATIENT, E.G. WHETHER
                    CURRENTLY IN HOSPITAL, WHETHER PNR OR
                    RNR,
              B30   NEW PNR/RNR IF THIS RECORD OBSOLETE.
              B15   DATE OF OBSOLESCENCE
             XB 2
              B 4   NON-ZERO = EXTRA CONFIDENTIAL
             XB 7
              B17   DEPT.
              B10   INSTN  RELATIVE TO VL RECORD
              B20   CLN
             XB 6
              B 9   PRELIM. ESTIMATE LENGTH OF DAY
              B15   PRELIM. ADMISSION DATE
              B10   CLN(WARD) IF CURRENTLY INPATIENT
              B20   INSTN
             XB 1
              B 6   NUMBER OF ADMISSION RECORDS IN P.R.
              B 6   NUMBER OF DISCHARGE RECORDS IN P.R.
              B17   DEPT IF CURRENTLY INPATIENT
              B15   PRELIM. DISCHARGE DATE
              B15   ADMISSION DATE
              C36   NAME
             XB 9
              B15   DATE OF LAST TRANSFER
              B15   FLAGS FOR USE OF CHEM. LAB. SUB-SYSTEM
             XB15   DATE
              B15   FLAGS FOR USE OF BOOKING SUB-SYSTEM
             XB 5
              B10   DEPT
             XB10
              B15   FLAGS
             XB 5
             XB10
             XC35
              B30   OLD PNR/RNR IF SUPERCEDING RECORD
              B30   LINK TO DBP RECORD
              B30   LINK TO VL RECORD
              B30   LINK TO SV RECORD
              B30   LINK TO OV RECORD
              B30   LINK TO KEM RECORD
```

TABLE 4-6. DATA DESCRIPTION OF HP FILE OF P.R.

(POCKET FILE, POCKET LENGTH = 429. ONE RECORD PER PATIENT.)

after the lead record, become disused by technical removal of their contents. At this point the ensemble is removed and the head record altered to show the pertinent sub-system file as inactive for the patient. If this sub-system was the last active for the patient, then the head record is marked as inactive, and thereby ultimately removed. (However, if a new event occurs before removal of the head record, the same record is re-activated.) Thus the P.R. acts as the repository for the accumulating history from an initial booking or emergency admission through to the completion of the case. Potentially this covers inpatient and outpatient services, but implementation of the latter is very restricted.

The inpatient file is the only component of the P.R. that has a direct correspondence with the Medical file of the H.R. However, while the latter has just one record per patient stay, the P.R. version has separate records

VL FILE

```
LEAD RECORD
               B 3   NON-ZERO = IN USE
               B12   NUMBER OF RECORDS (MAX 99)
               B15   NUMBER OF WORDS IN ENSEMBLE (MAX 99)
               B30   PNR/RNR
               B10   CLN (WARD) IN WHICH BOOKED
               B20   INSTN
               C 1   ACCOMMODATION-TYPE REQUIRED (AC)
               C 1   PRIORITY (PRTY)
              XB 1
               B17   DEPT
              XB 1
               B 9   ESTIMATED LENGTH OF STAY
               B 4   EXPECTED ADMISSION CODE (ADMC)
               B 1   1 = TO BE ADMITTED FROM O.P. DEPT.
               B15   PRELIM. ADMISSION DATE
               B 1   1 = STANDARD ADMISSION TESTS REQUIRED
              XB 2
              XB 7
               B20   INSTN REFERRING PATIENT
               C 2   NATIONALITY
              XB 1
               B17   DEPT REFERRING PATIENT
              XB11
               B 4   CIVIL STATUS
               B15   DATE IN WHICH BOOKING WAS MADE
               C27   STREET ADDRESS
               B 1 = SPECIAL CONFIDENTIALITY
               B17   POST CODE
               C13   POST TOWN
               C12   TELEPHONE NUMBER
               C10   PROFESSION/OCCUPATION
              XB30
GENERAL RECORD (COMMON FIELDS). NO OCCURRENCE
               B 9   RECORD TYPE CODE
               B 9   NUMBER OF WORDS IN RECORD
ONE RECORD (SPECIAL TESTS UPON ADMISSION). OCCURS 0-1
               B18   SEE GENERAL RECORD (RECORD TYPE = 001)
               C40   SPECIAL TESTS TO BE PERFORMED
TWO RECORD (ANCILLARY PROCEDURES). OCCURS 0-3
               B18   SEE GENERAL RECORD (RECORD TYPE = 002)
               C 3   TERMINAL OPERATOR'S INITIALS
              XB 4
               B20   CODE FOR PROCEDURE
              XB15
               B15   DATE
               C25   PROCEDURE, BY NAME.
THREE RECORD (ALTERATION OF PRELIM. ADM. DATE)
               B18   SEE GENERAL RECORD (RECORD TYPE = 003)
              XB 8
               B 4   1 = PATNT REQUEST; 2 = HOSP REQUEST
               B15   OLD DATE
               B15   REVISED DATE
FOUR RECORD (DIAGNOSIS). OCCURS 0-3.
               B18   SEE GENERAL RECORD (RECORD TYPE = 004)
               C17   PRELIM. DIAGNOSIS
```

TABLE 4-7. DATA DESCRIPTION OF VL FILE OF P.R.

(LINKED FILE. PATIENT RECORD-ENSEMBLE VARIES FROM 22 TO 999 WORDS, AVERAGE SIZE 37 WORDS.)

SV FILE

```
LEAD RECORD
          B 3   NON-ZERO = IN USE
          B12   NUMBER OF RECORDS (MAX 100)
          B15   NUMBER  OF  WORDS  IN  RECORD-ENSEMBLE
                (MAX 999)
          B30   PNR/RNR
          C27   STREET ADDRESS
         XB 1
          B17   POSTAL CODE
          C13   POST TOWN
          C 2   NAT
          C36   NEXT OF KIN'S NAME
          B 7   MUNICIPALITY OF RESIDENCE
          C27   NEXT OF KIN'S STREET ADDRESS
          B 4   CIVIL STATUS
          B14   BRANCH NUMBER OF STATE INSUR. OFFICE.
          C13   NEXT OF KIN'S POST TOWN
          C 2   COUNTY OF RESIDENCE (NUMBER)
          C10   PROFESSION/OCCUPATION
          C12   NEXT OF KIN'S TELEPHONE NUMBER
GENERAL RECORD (COMMON FIELDS). NO OCCURRENCE
          B 9   RECORD TYPE CODE
          B 9   NUMBER OF WORDS IN RECORD
ISV RECORD (ADMISSION)
          B18   SEE GENERAL RECORD (RECORD TYPE = 001)
          B15   DATE OF ADMISSION
          B 7   CONTROL FLAGS
          B10   DEPT OF CURRENT LOCATION
          B10   CLN (WARD)
          C 1   ADMC (ADMISSION CODE)
         XB 1
          B 3   NUMBER OF DIAGNOSES (GROUP 1)
          B20   INSTN OF CURRENT LOCATION
          B 1   CORRECTED   FIELD,   TO   BE   ADVISED
                ERRONEOUS DATA REPORTED TO FSK
          B 7   PCL, PATIENT CLASS
          B 1   NON-ZERO = EMERGENCY ADMISSION
          B 1   NON-ZERO = ADMITTED FROM O.P. CLINIC
          B 4   NON-ZERO = ADMISSION CODE
          B 2   PART-TIME INPATIENT
          B 1   1 = NAME TO BE OBSCURED EXTRA CONFINED
         XB 3
          B10   DEPT THAT REFERRED CASE
          B 1   NON-ZERO = REPORTED TO STATE INSUR OFF
          B 9   ESTIMATED LENGTH OF STAY
          B20   INSTN THAT REFERRED CASE
     GROUP 1 : DIAGNOSES
          C17   DIAGNOSIS (TEXT)
         XC 3
USV RECORD (DISCHARGE)
          B18   SEE GENERAL RECORD (RECORD TYPE = 002)
          B15   DATE OF DISCHARGE
          B 7   CONTROL FLAGS
          B10   DEPT FROM WHICH DISCHARGED
          B10   CLN (WARD)
          B 1   1 = ONE E-CODE, 0 = NONE
          B 4   NUMBER OF DIAGNOSES (GROUP 2)
          B 1   1 = DISCHARGED TO OUTPATIENT CLINIC
          B 4   DISC (DISCHARGE CODE)
         XB 1
          B 3   RESULTS OF T.B. VARIOUS TESTS
          B 1   NON-ZERO  =  T.B. (1 = NEWLY DIAG, 2 =
                OLD CASE)
          B14   INSTN FROM WHICH DISCHARGED
          B 1   NON-ZERO = REPORTED TO STATE INSUR OFF
          B12   TIME OF DISCHARGE, AT LEAST FOR DEATHS
         XB 7
          B10   DEPT TO WHICH DISCHARGED (IF ANY)
          B 8   NUMBER OF DAYS WITH LEAVE OF ABSENCE
          B 1   NON-ZERO  =  REPORTED  ERRONEOUSLY  TO
                STATE INSURANCE OFFICE.
         XB 3
          B 4   NUMBER OF E CODES (GROUP 1)
```

```
          B14   INSTN TO WHICH DISCHARGED (IF ANY)
      GROUP 1 : TYPE OF ACCIDENT ETC.
          C 5   E CODE (I.E. CAUSE OF ILL-HEALTH)
      GROUP 2 : DIAGNOSES
          C 5   DIAGNOSIS (ICDC)
          B 1   NON-ZERO = CAUSE OF DEATH
          B14   OPERATION (OPNC)
          B15   OPERATION DATE
          B 4   DAY NUMBER OF OPERATION
         XB 9
          B17   ANAESTHESIA CODE
PIK RECORD (TRANSFER TO/FROM TECHNICAL DEPT.)
          B18   SEE GENERAL RECORD (RECORD TYPE = 002)
          B15   DATE OF TRANSFER
          B17   TECHNICAL DEPT
          B10   CLN (WARD) THEREIN
          B12   TIME OF TRANSFER
         XB 5
          B 3   TYPE  OF TRANSFER (1 = PIK DIALOG, 2 =
                TTA, 3 = FTA)
          B10   CLN (WARD) OF NORMAL DEPT.
PP RECORD (LEAVE OF ABSENCE)
          B18   SEE GENERAL RECORD (RECORD TYPE = 004)
          B15   DATE OF START OF ABSENCE
          B17   DEPT FROM WHICH ABSENT
          B10   CLN (WARD)
         XB 3
          B12   TIME OF START OF ABSENCE
          B15   DATE OF RETURN FROM ABSENCE (APPROVED)
         XB14
          B 4   REASON FOR ABSENCE (LOAC)
          B12   TIME OF RETURN FROM ABSENCE (APPROVED)
PU RECORD (EXPECTED DISCHARGE)
         XB18   SEE GENERAL RECORD (RECORD TYPE = 005)
          B15   DATE
          B17   DEPT OF ORIGINATION OF ESTIMATE
          B10   CLN (WARD)
          B15   DATE EXPECTED FOR DISCHARGE
         XB15
KU RECORD (RELEASE FOR DISCHARGE)
         XB18   SEE GENERAL RECORD (RECORD TYPE = 006)
          B15   DATE
          B17   DEPT WHEN RELEASE MADE
          B10   CLN (WARD)
          B15   DATE FOR RECALL, IF ANY
          B15   DATE WHEN DISCHARGE CAN OCCUR
         XB 9
          B 4   INTENDED DISC (DISCHARGE CODE)
          B17   DEPT PROPOSED  FOR  DISCHARGE  TO  (IF
                ANY)
         XB10
          B20   INSTN  PROPOSED  FOR  DISCHARGE TO (IF
                ANY)
```

TABLE 4-8. DATA DESCRIPTION OF SV FILE OF P.R.

(LINKED FILE. PATIENT RECORD-ENSEMBLE FROM 33 TO 999 WORDS; AVERAGE SIZE 95 TO 190 WORDS.)

DBP FILE

```
LEAD RECORD
          B 3   NON-ZERO = IN USE
          B12   NUMBER OF RECORDS (MAX 200)
          B15   NUMBER OF WORDS IN RECORD-ENSEMBLE
                (MAX 999)
          B30   PNR/RNR
          B10   ORDINAL OF FIRST FREE SUB-RECORD
          B 2
         XB18
GENERAL RECORD (COMMON FIELDS). NO OCCURRENCE.
          B 9   RECORD TYPE CODE
          B 9   NUMBER OF WORDS IN RECORD
                BOOKING WITHIN BOOKING ORDER
          B10   BOOKING ORDER NUMBER
          B 1   NON-ZERO = ERRONEOUS SUB-RECORD
          B 1   NON-ZERO = NON-CURRENT SUB-RECORD
BEST RECORD (ONE PER BOOKING ORDER)
          B30   SEE GENERAL RECORD (RECORD TYPE = 001)
          B15   DATE OF RECORDING BOOKING
          B 3   NUMBER OF COMMENTS (GROUP )
          C12   REFERENCE NOTE
          B20   INSTN BY WHICH BOOKING MADE
          B10   DEPT BY WHICH BOOKING MADE
         XB 5
          B17   CLN BY WHICH BOOKING MADE
     GROUP 1 : COMMENT
          B14   EXTERNAL EXAMINATION CODE
         XB 4
          C22   COMMENT
UND RECORD      (ONE PER BOOKING)
          B30   SEE GENERAL RECORD (RECORD TYPE = 002)
          B14   RESOURCE CODE
          B15   DATE OF SERVICE
         XB 1
          B 8   START TIME
          B 8   FINISH TIME       EXPRESSED AS MULTIPLE
          B 8   ARRIVAL TIME      OF 5 MINS. AFTER
                                  07:00
          B 8   DEPARTURE TIME    HRS.
          B14   EXAM
          B10   DEPT PROVIDING SERVICE
          B 2   NON-ZERO = PATIENT NOT SEEN (E.G. 3 =
                PATIENT ABSENT ILL)
          B 2   INDICATES WHETHER NOTICE PRINTED FOR
                PATIENT
```

TABLE 4-9. DATA DESCRIPTION OF DBP FILE OF P.R. (LINKED FILE. PATIENT RECORD-ENSEMBLE 7 TO 999 WORDS; AVERAGE SIZE 32 TO 42 WORDS.)

OV FILE

```
LEAD RECORD
          B 3   NON-ZERO = IN USE
          B12   NUMBER OF RECORDS (MAX 33)
          B15   NUMBER OF WORDS IN RECORD-ENSEMBLE
                (MAX 4092)
          B30   PNR/RNR
          B14   STATE INSURANCE BRANCH (NON-RESIDENTS
                OF COUNTY ONLY)
GENERAL RECORD (COMMON FIELDS). NO OCCURRENCE
          B 9   RECORD TYPE CODE
          B 9   NUMBER OF WORDS IN RECORD
          B17   DEPT FOR SERVICE
          B 6   NUMBER OF OCCURRENCES OF GROUP 1.
OPVM RECORD (SEQUENCE OF VISITS)
          B41   SEE GENERAL RECORD (RECORD TYPE = 001)
          B 7   TOTAL VISITS TO THIS POINT
          B20   INSTN REFERRING PATIENT
          B17   DEPT REFERRING PATIENT
          B 3   REFERENCE FROM 1 = OUTPATIENT CLINIC,
                2 = INPATIENT, ETC.
          B 3   REFERRED TO 1 = OWN INPATIENT SERVICE
                2 = OTHER DEPT., ETC.
          B20   INSTN REFERRED TO
          B17   DEPT REFERRED TO
          B 1   0 = COMPLETE HERE; 1 = FURTHER VISIT
          B 2   INSULIN TREATMENT
          B 2   ANTI-COAGULANT TREATMENT
          B 2   CORTISONE TREATMENT
         XB 1
          B15   START DATE FOR SICK NOTE
          B15   STOP DATE FOR SICK NOTE
         XB14
     GROUP 1
          B 3   TYPE OF VISIT (1 = NEW, 2 = RETURN, 3
                = INDIRECT).
          B15   VISIT DATE
          B 1   1 = EMERGENCY ATTENDANCE
          B 7   LOCATION WITHIN HOSPITAL. (RECEPTION)
          B17   DOCTOR, BY CODE NUMBER
          B 2   SICK NOTE; 0 = NO, 1 = FULL, 2 =
                PARTIAL
          B 2   VISIT RESULT; 0 = BETTER, 1 =
                UNCHANGED, 2 = WORSE
          B 1   1 = DIAGNOSIS STILL UNDER
                INVESTIGATION
          B 1   1 = A DIAGNOSIS RECORDED
          B17   ANAESTHESIA CODE
          C 5   FIRST DIAGNOSIS (ICDC)
          C 5   SECOND DIAGNOSIS (ICDC)
          B14   FIRST PROCEDURE (CODE)
          B14   SECOND PROCEDURE (CODE)
          B14   OPERATION CODE
          B 7   VACCINATIONS AND SERUM TREATMENTS
          B 7   VACCINATIONS AND SERUM TREATMENTS
          B 7   VACCINATIONS AND SERUM TREATMENTS
          C 8   DRUG WITH ADVERSE SIDE EFFECT
          B 2   NUMBER OF CONTERMATION GROUPS
          B 1   WHETHER THIS OR CURRENT
         XC15
```

TABLE 4-10. DATA DESCRIPTION OF OV FILE OF P.R.

(LINKED FILE. PATIENT RECORD-ENSEMBLE 24 TO 999 WORDS; AVERAGE SIZE 58 TO 63 WORDS).

<u>KEM</u> <u>FILE</u>

```
LEAD RECORD
          B 3   NON-ZERO = IN USE
          B12   NUMBER OF RECORDS (MAX 297)
          B15   NUMBER OF WORDS IN ENSEMBLE (MAX 4092)
          B30   PNR/RNR
          B15   DATE OF LAST ENTRY TO RECORD-ENSEMBLE
         XB11
          B 1   1 = INFECTIVE
          B 1   1 = HEPATETIC
          B 1   1 = AT LEAST ONE REQUISITION ON HAND
          B 1   1 = NEW RESULT SINCE LAST LAB LIST
         XC15
GENERAL RECORD
          B 9   RECORD TYPE CODE
          B 9   NUMBER OF WORDS IN RECORD
UB RECORD (RESULTS ) IN REVERSE CHRONOLOGICAL ORDER.
          B18   SEE GENERAL RECORD (RECORD TYPE = 001)
          B12   NUMBER OF TESTS (GROUP 1)
          B15   DATE OF TAKING SPECIMEN
          B15   SPECIMEN NUMBER
          B18   INSTN
          B12   DEPT  REQUISITIONING
          B18   CLN (WARD)
          B12   TIME  OF  TAKING  SPECIMEN  (WHERE
                SIGNIF.)
          B18   REQUISITIONING DOCTOR (CODE)
          B 6   PATIENT CATEGORY
          B 6   NUMBER OF COMMENTS (GROUP 2)
          B 3   SPECIMEN NUMBER CANCELLED UNLESS 0
          B 3   SPECIMEN NR AFFIXED BY LAB. COMPUTER
         XB18
          B 6   CONTROL FLAGS
     GROUP 1 : RESULTS           (1-120)
          B15   TEST CODE
          B 6   COMMENT NR (I.E. OCCURRENCE OF GRP 2)
         XB 3
          B 6   CONTROL FLAGS
          C 5   TEST RESULT
     GROUP 2 : COMMENT           (0-63)
          C80   COMMENT
PB RECORD (REQUISITION) IN ASCENDING CHRON ORDER
          B18   SEE GENERAL RECORD (RECORD TYPE = 002)
          B12   TIME OF BOOKING
          B 9   NUMBER OF TESTS REQUISITIONED
          B 6   LOCATION
          B15   DATE  OF SPECIMEN-DRAWING
          B12   TIME
          B18   INSTN
          B12   DEPT
          B18   CLN (WARD)
          B18   DOCTOR (CODE)
          B12   ROOM & BED
          B12   TIME FOR TIME-LIMITED ANSWER
         XB14
          B 1   0 = OUTPATIENT, 1 = INPATIENT.
          B 3   PATNT CAT 0 = INP 1 = OUTP 2 = ADM
         XB30
     GROUP 1
          B15   TEST CODE
          B 3   ANSWER (2 = PHONE, 4 = TIME LMTT)
         XB11
          B 1   1 = CANCELLED
```

<u>TABLE</u> 4-11. DATA DESCRIPTION OF KEM FILE OF P.R.

(LINKED FILE. PATIENT RECORD ENSEMBLE 15 TO 4092 WORDS; AVERAGE SIZE 220 TO 300 WORDS).

for admisssion and discharge, plus records for every transfer and leave of absence that occur. Special records are also provided, as Table 4-8 shows, for provisional and firm notice of impending discharge. Added to the lead record, such a variety of records covers each stay currently in the P.R., one set being succeeded by another where appropriate.

Removal of information from the P.R. to the H.R., as happens with the inpatient synopsis, and more generally to off-line archival storage, is effected by batch programs that are executed once a day at most, and much less often mostly. Hence, there can be a significant amount of completed data held in a P.R. at any particular instant.

The P.R.s - Volume of data

The operational practices regarding removal of completed records, particularly to the archival storage, the policy regarding minimum retention period on the P.R., and even the hospitals' practices in regard to length in advance that bookings are made, all influence the amount of data in the P.R.s, beyond the more basic influences of hospital sizes and degree of sub-system implementation. The policy of retaining inpatient records for 30 days after discharge implies the number of inpatient stays being a minimum of four times the inpatient capacity for general hospitals. Retention for outpatient records in the P.R. is currently set as a minimum of 90 days.

P.R.	#1	#2	#3	#4	#5	#6	#7	#8	#9	ALL
HEAD RECORDS	53,067	1,951	3,141	2,155	2,914	8,897	14,721	2,724	9,384	98,954
OVERFLOW	5,220	74	57	44	0	0	0	0	188	5,583
%	9.8%	3.79%	1.8%	2.0	0.0	0.0	0.0	0.0	2.0	5.6%
VL ENSEMBLES	49,081				3	3.639		747	1,713	55,183
%	92.5%				0.1	40.9%		27.4%	18.3%	55.8%
SV ENSEMBLES	4.944	1,951	3,141	2,155	1,733	6,260	14,721	2,439	8,160	45,504
%	9.32%	100.0	100.0	100%	59.5%	70.4%	100.0	89.5%	86.96%	46.0%
DBP ENSEMBLES	5,109					2,481			1,159	8,749
	9.63%					27.9%			12.4%	8.8%
OV ENSEMBLES	46,260									46,260
%	87.2%									46.8%
KEM ENSEMBLES	16,495				2,770					19,265
%	31.1%				95.1%					19.5%
BED TOTAL	787	437	673	543	1,519	1,061	1,346	548	1,776	8,690

TABLE 4-12. NUMBERS OF RECORD-ENSEMBLES IN P.R. FILES.

% MEANS PERCENTAGE OF HEAD RECORDS
P.R.#1 = HUDDINGE, P.R.#2 = NACKA, P.R.#3 = SABBATSBERG, P.R.#4 = ST. ERIK'S, P.R.#5 = BECKOMBERGA, P.R.#6 = DANDERYD, P.R.#7 = SODER, P.R.#8 = SODERTALJE, P.R.#9 = KAROLINSKA

Table 4-12 gives, for each of the nine P.R.s currently established, statistics on the number of patients in each of the constituent files, together with the number of beds covered by each P.R. The long-term psychiatric hospital at Beckomberga (P.R. #5), with its greater average length of stay, has a proportionally low number of inpatient record-ensembles, but elsewhere the number of such ensembles is mostly of the order of five times the bed number. Distinctive retention practices for Soder hospital (#7) lead to this large hospital having over ten times the bed number for its active inpatient total. The nine P.R.s average 11 000 patients each, but nearly half of this figure is attributable to the outpatient application at Huddinge. Neglecting these and the special case of Beckomberga, the average is 5 400 patients relative to 900 beds.

The erratic proportion of head records that overflow is attributable to both discrepancies between anticipated and actual populations and to the restriction - only recently removed - to one standard figure for file size. Adjustment of the number of pockets is not simply made and must, therefore, bear in mind both current gain and future demand. The standard size adopted for the first five hospitals has proved too small for Huddinge but large to excessive for the other four, which have the zero overflows.

The provision of disk space for the sub-system files has also been rather varied compared with related needs, but has recently been adjusted after the major phase of implementation. The actual space required for these files builds up progressively between the occasions when the completed records are removed and, simultaneously, the remaining records are repacked. The range of size per record-ensemble is shown in the footnote to each of the Tables 4-7 thru 4-11. The reduction process is currently executed every two weeks, on alternating halves of the relevant file set. Table 4-16, later in this chapter, shows the space required immediately before and after the compaction step, for several representative files, including the largest P.R. files - those for Huddinge hospital.

The long-term trend for P.R. files should, unlike the Medical file set of the H.R., be stable. However, both long- and short-term patterns are watched continually through a daily report on actual file occupation.

V.R. - THE WAITING LIST

V.R. - organization

Although at one time envisioned as a sub-system file of the P.R., the collection of records of patients awaiting service could not be divided by institution without impairing the integrated planning basis of the application. Hence the waiting list is outside of the P.R. data files, and has its own distinctive definition. However, its organization is again one of pocket file plus linked file, the latter related to the fact that a patient can be waiting for more than one service (a fact all the more true in this System by its inclusion of many outpatient services in those covered by the waiting list).

The specification for the head record is in Table 4-13, where it can be seen that RNR is again an allowable alternative to PNR. The record comprises typical contact data, plus one link address, and occupies one segment. Pocket size is 12 segments, and 4 463 pockets are used. Current population of the list is around 31 000.

HEAD FILE

```
HEAD RECORD                          (LENGTH 33 WORDS)
        B30   PNR/RNR
        B30   BIRTHDATE (RNR CASE)
        B 1   1 = DEPARTED FROM COUNTY
        B 1   1 = REMOVED FROM H.R.
        B 1   1 = RECORD TO BE RETAINED DESPITE
              DEPARTURE
       XB 2
        B 1   1 = RECORD STILL ACTIVE
        C36   PATIENT'S NAME (SURNAME, FORENAMES)
       XB 1
        B17   POST CODE
        C10   PROFESSION/OCCUPATION
        C27   STREET ADDRESS
        C13   POST TOWN
        C12   TELEPHONE NUMBER (HOME)
       XB18
        B30   LINK TO ASSOCIATED RECORD
        C12   TELEPHONE NUMBER (WORK)
       XC33
```

TABLE 4-13. DATA DESCRIPTION OF HEAD FILE OF V.R.

(POCKET FILE; POCKET SIZE = 429 WORDS, 4463 POCKETS).

Table 4-14 provides the specification of the associated linked file (VPL). Following the same control and identification as in the previous linked files, the specification allows up to 10 records for separate independent demands, each itself having a degree of variability through the existence of optional groups at its end. The fields included provide for expression of priority and urgency as well as need, and allow for updating as booking occurs.

As with the sub-system files of the P.R., the individual patient's ensemble here can have records subtracted from it as well as added, so appropriate marking must be provided on each.

V.R. - population and size

The V.R. has a population of about 31 000, which is markedly less than the 40 000 to 45 000 anticipated when the file was established. Consequently the pockets, designed on the usual 12-records, 80%-utility criteria, have a nominal utility of only around 60%. The specification of a 33-word record, which entails a whole segment per pocket for the overflow link field, has built in another 7% loss in utilization, leaving practical utilization of the space assigned to the head file at barely 50%. Overflow is correspondingly small, bringing the total disk-space assignment for head records to 2.1 million words.

About 3.5 million words are currently assigned to the linked file; with an average size of about 70 words per record-ensemble the utilization is of the order of 60%. However, as with the P.R. sub-system files, there is a 'saw-tooth' pattern to the space-needs of this file; Table 4-15 shows the figures before and after one monthly compaction.

VPL FILE (RECORD LENGTH ? TO 594 WORDS)

```
LEAD RECORD
        B 3   NON-ZERO = IN USE
        B12   NUMBER OF RECORDS (MAX 10)
        B15   NUMBER OF WORDS IN RECORD-ENSEMBLE
              (MAX 594)
        B30   PNR/RNR
GENERAL RECORD (COMMON FIELDS). NO OCCURRENCE
        B 9   RECORD TYPE CODE
        B 9   NUMBER OF WORDS IN RECORD
DEMAND RECORD. OCCURS 1 TO 9.
        B18   SEE GENERAL RECORD (RECORD TYPE = 001)
        B 2   NUMBER OF DEMAND
        B 1
        B 1
        B 2   STATUS FLAG (1 = NEW SINCE LAST
              LISTING, 2 = CHANGED CODES)
        B 1   STATUS CONTROL FLAG1 (1 = ADDITION
              SINCE LAST LISTING)
        B 2   STATUS CONTROL FLAG2 (1 = CANCELLATION
              SINCE LAST LISTING)
        B 9   DAY (OF YEAR) OF ENTRY
        B 2   TYPE OF ACCOMMODATION REQUIRED (AC)
        B 3   COMPLETION CODE (1 = ADMITTED AS A
              COSTS CASE, 2 = ADMITTED ROUTINELY, 3
              = DECEASED, 4 = OTHER REASON FOR
              CANCELLATION, 5 = ERRONEOUS ENTRY)
        B20   INSTN (DESIRED)
        B15   DATE OF REGISTRATION  ALL EXPRESSED
        B15   DATE OF AMENDING      RELATIVE TO
        B15   PLANNED ADM. DATE     1960, IN YEARS
        B15   CRITICAL DATE         THEN DAYS.
        B17   DEPT CONCERNED
        B 5   PROPOSED DAY, RELATIVE TO ADMISSION,
              FOR OPERATION
        B 2   REFERRED FROM 0 = EMERGENCY, 1 =
              INPATIENT 2 = OUTPATIENT, 3 = FROM
              HOME.
        B 1   0 = INPATIENT SERVICE 2 = OUTPATIENT
              SERVICE
        B 6   YEAR OF REGISTRATION (RELATIVE TO
              1960)
        B 1   1 = REGISTERED BY ISV DIALOG
        B 7   DEPARTMENTAL PLANNING CODE
        B 3   PRTY
        C 3
        B15   DATE OF CANCELLATION
        B14   OPERATION CODE
        B 1   1 = PATIENT INFECTED
    GROUP 1 (REFERRING DOCTOR) OCCURS 0 TO 1
        C20   DOCTOR'S NAME
    GROUP 2 (NOTE ) OCCURS 0 TO 1
        C10   REFERRING CIRCUMSTANCES
    GROUP 3 (DIAGNOSIS) OCCURS 0 TO 3
        C15   DIAGNOSIS (TEXT)
        C20   COMMENT
        C 5   DIAGNOSIS (ICDC)
```

TABLE 4-14. DATA DESCRIPTION OF VPL FILE OF V.R.

(LINKED FILE. PATIENT RECORD ENSEMBLE 50 TO 594 WORDS; AVERAGE SIZE 60 TO 80 WORDS.)

FILE	SIZE OF FILE 11FEB76	16FEB76	13MAR76	15MAR76	SPACE ASSIGNED
HS PR HP*	2529582	2525820	2591490	2522490	2640000
HS PR VL	1786686	1731741	1858461	1783320	1921920
HS PR SV	597267	477576	672903	510642	707267
HS PR BOK	210078	170808	242319	172821	316800
HS PR OV	2902218	2657094	3035637	2749989	3125760
HS PR KEM	3793185	3126024	4235517	3225816	5280000
HS KEM009	594396	580668	616516	606276	1501632
SE PR HP*	234432	232122	235092	232782	266112
SE PR SV	388971	210 573	303534	218196	650496
VR HP*	1963137	1973433	2 055669	2007093	2112000
VR VPL	2508528	1825131	2168826	1754775	3484800

TABLE 4-15. FLUCTUATING SIZE OF SOME MAJOR FILES

'HS' AND 'SE' REFER TO HUDDINGE AND ST. ERIK'S HOSPITALS, BEING COLUMNS #1 AND #4 RESPECTIVELY IN PRECEDING TABLES.
* INDICATES POCKET FILES, FOR WHICH THE STATED SIZE INCLUDES ALL SPACE ASSIGNED TO POCKETS; THE FLUCTUATION AND RESIDUAL FREE SPACE PERTAINS ONLY TO THE OVERFLOW COMPONENT OF ASSIGNED SPACE.
EACH OF THE PAIRS OF COLUMNS COVERS A WEEKEND DURING WHICH STRIPPING AND PACKING OF THESE FILES OCCURRED. HOWEVER, THE FIRST COLUMN RELATES TO THE THURSDAY, AND AS ALL COLUMNS ARE EARLY MORNING OBSERVATIONS, THIS ALLOWS TWO DAYS' FURTHER ACCUMULATION BEFORE REDUCTION.

OTHER ON-LINE FILES

Outside of the program modules and certain data they embed, the on-line data base includes:-

Clear Text files for translating codes into clear text and, in most cases, checking the acceptability of input text and effecting the coding for storage.

Resource files, providing catalogs of the services provided and of the resources that provide them, and keeping record of their commitment and availability.

Laboratory Analyses files, providing a catalog of the available tests, augmented by their textural descriptions and their normal value ranges.

Care files, relating operations and other primary procedures to the tests and other ancillary procedures that should be routinely associated with them, and acting as repositories for their observed statistics regarding length-of-stay, duration of operation, etc.

In all these files the information is stored in generalized modules, retrievable and if necessary restructured by generalized data base programs. The Resource files, which, like the Laboratory Analyses files, are in separate data files for each pertinent institution, are effectively on-line master files for the booking application, and must be updated as regards commitments in real-time mode. Otherwise these files are of more of a reference-only nature for the real-time processes.

STORAGE OF ON-LINE FILES

Table 4-16 gives a summary of the amount of disk storage assigned to the on-line files. Of the total 188.7 million words, virtually a half is for the H.R. About 36 million words are required for the P.R.s, but the booking, outpatient and chemical laboratory sub-systems add significantly to the file storage required for each hospital in which they are implemented. For the one hospital with all three - Huddinge - this adds about 60% to the storage required for the V.R. alone, a requirement that is itself inflated by the same sub-systems.

	P.R.S AND OTHER HOSPITAL-SEGREGATED FILES									H.R.	V.R.	OTHER
	1	2	3	4	5	6	7	8	9			
HEAD FILES	2.6	0.2	0.3	0.3	2.2	2.2	2.2	2.2	0.0	45.8	2.1	
LINKED FILES	11.3	0.5	0.7	0.7	3.0	1.5	1.8	0.8	2.5	45.0	3.5	
ASSOC. FILES	9.8	0.1	0.1	0.1	1.5	1.3	0.1	0.1	1.6	3.0	0.1	38.8
TOTALS	23.7	0.8	1.1	1.1	6.7	5.0	4.1	3.1	5.0			
TOTALS					50.6					93.8	5.7	38.8

TABLE 4-16. DISPOSITION OF ASSIGNED DISK STORAGE.

'HEAD FILES' COVERS THE POCKET FILES DESCRIBED, AND THEIR OVERFLOW AREAS
'LINKED FILES' COVERS THE LINKED FILES DESCRIBED
'ASSOC. FILES' COVERS FILES NOT DESCRIBED IN DETAIL IN CHAPTER 4
'OTHER' COVERS COMMON DATA FILES OTHER THAN H.R. & V.R., PLUS TEXT FILES AND VARIOUS SYSTEM-CONTROL FILES.
SEE TABLE 4-12 FOR INTERPRETATION OF COLUMN-HEADING NUMBERS.

The disk capacity of the central computing equipment is 327 million words. Each of the three '8460' units that provide this capacity functions as two logically separated entitities; hence the capacity may be seen as 6 units of 54.5 million words each. To allow easy relocation of files in case of breakdown, and in fact to allow preventive maintenance, the real-time production files are restricted to a sub-set of these six. The current demand of 188.7 million words allows restriction to four logical units, leaving one available for the substantial testing that continuing development demands, as well as one out of use.

The on-line files are therefore assembled into four groups, to a maximum of 54.5 million words each. In deciding the particulars of assembly, effort is made to balance the access-demand loads of the four groups, rather than their sizes, which are

Group A 44.3 million words
Group B 52.1 million words
Group C 44.7 million words
Group D 47.8 million words

Within each group the placement of files is made with a view to reducing the average access time, by placing the files that have a lower intensity of access at the two extremes and the busier files in the middle of the group. The largest file - the Adult CFU file - occupies 36.4 million words alone, so must occupy the middle area irrespective of its exact placement. However, such a necessity has been avoided for the infrequently accessed, 45 million words, of Medical file data, by the artificial division into individual files of 5 million words each.

The total file set is re-assembled monthly or so, when new files are cataloged into the system and existing files are adjusted in size or place as appropriate. If any inadequacy of space assignment emerges between re-assembles, an additional area can be connected logically to the particular file as a stop-gap measure, even during real-time processing.

To assist planning of the arrangement of these files, a detailed study of accessing traffic is conducted annually.

OFF-LINE FILES

Besides the very many files belonging to other fields from health care using Datacentral, there are three important sets of files for health care maintained on magnetic tape, namely

- Health Control and Home Care Files containing information on examinations and tests to be performed, on results of tests and analyses, and on ordered therapies - in relation to home care and health control.
- Statistics files containing selected information from the P.R.s and from the above tape files, sufficiently more detailed than the H.R. to allow some use as synopses of individual patient care but more generally for statistical analyses and planning.
- Patient History Files, being the archival repository for virtually all P.R. data.

In addition to the above, logs are kept on magnetic tape of each contact with the computer through a terminal, and of the 'before' and 'after' status of every real-time update.

Beside the computer-legible files and the orthodox manual records that necessarily remain to a considerable degree, the overall medical information system involves microfiche records. The most notable example is with x-rays, with the pictures and report of every examination in the County being recorded on microfiche and thereby made available to all x-ray departments. The RTG record of the H.R. provides the briefest summary of each case, and gives the necessary pointer to the microfiche.

CHAPTER 5

ACCESSING THE DATA BASE

It is clear from the foregoing chapter that, though the H.R. has a central function across all applications, it is the V.R., for the waiting list sub-system, and the P.R.s, for the other four, with which the sub-systems essentially function. For non-residents at least, the latter four deal only with the one P.R. pertaining to the institution concerned, plus resource or reference files involved, and no sub-system involves the H.R. in any way. Even within a P.R., the relationship of any one syb-system is only with a selection of files, at most three of the six. The relationship of the primary applicational sub-systems to the data base is illustrated in Fig 5-1; with them are illustrated also two minor functions outside of the particular sub-system - the retrieval of H.R. information for an identified person and the search for PERSON-NUMB.

Though the on-line data base can be accessed through off-line means (this, for instance, being the only means for updating the H.R.), and on-line access can be gained via teleprinters, it is the c.r.t. upon which the System depends for real-time operations. Though there are three different models in use, they are all very similar and the system features and practices established with the early Uniscope terminals remain essentially unchanged with the Alfascope that now comprises a majority of the over 200 terminals in use. Chapter 3 has described the terminal network and given an outline of terminals. However, to understand the operational System requires some expansion on that earlier description and some explanation of the standard practices adopted for this System. This starts most appropriately with a look at the Alfascope as equipment, then proceeds to the manner of use adopted.

THE ALFASCOPE

The Alfascope as equipment

The Stansaab Alfascope terminal consists of a c.r.t. display unit plus cable-connected keyboard, with refresh memory and raster generation in a controller that handles up to eight terminals. A multiplexing bus allows up to eight controllers to share one line. Any terminal slot can be occupied instead by a printer (or other compatible device), while printers can, and often are, connected to controllers in parallel with terminals - able to take the data direct from the c.r.t.'s memory.

Except for the three additional characters of the Swedish alphabet, the keyboard, which is illustrated in Fig 5-2, is of a familiar appearance. Appendix C provides a specification of the keys which, beside the alphanumeric key set plus a 10-key numeric section, include

- 12 edit keys for cursor control, erasing, deletion and insertion of embedded data, new line, repetition and tabulation
- 6 function keys for clear screen, reset keyboard, calling for display of unsolicited output message, initiation of local printing, initiation of transmission, and blinking of a word on the screen
- 5 program keys that each cause transmission of a fixed sequence of

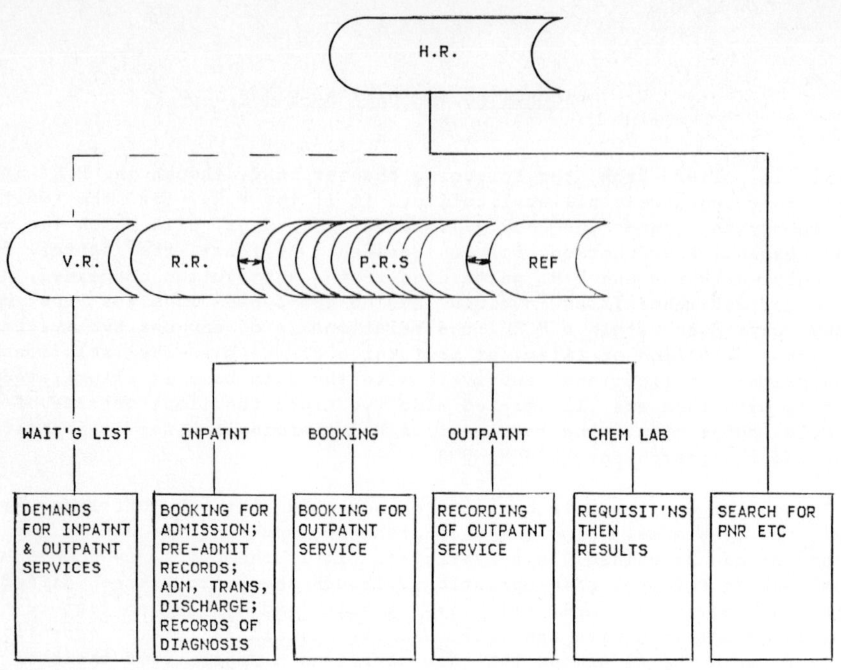

<u>FIG</u> 5-1 RELATIONSHIP OF MAJOR FILES AND SUB-SYSTEMS

R.R. = RESOURCE FILE REF = REFERENCE FILE
SHORT-DASHED LINES INDICATE REFERENCE ONLY
LONG-DASHED LINES INDICATE OFF-LINE UPDATING
CONTINUOUS LINES INDICATE ON-LINE UPDATING

characters.

The screen contains 17 rows of 64 characters each, of which the last row is usable only as display related to the function keys, leaving 1024 positions for data purposes. The visible non-destructive cursor can be moved explicitly up or down, to left or right, or directly to the 'home' position at the top left of the screen. It is moved automatically as any character is entered in its place. It passes between the last position of row 17 and the home position as though they were consecutive.

Transmission of data between terminal and computer can relate to a part only of the screen, leaving the remainder untouched; the part can start and end at any position on the screen. Specification within the message of the start position other than home position is made using the ESCape feature of the ASCII coding scheme, with two characters representing the row/column matrix position. This special character sequence, ended by the SI character, is placed immediately following the STX character. Variable-length-text provisions in the messages allow for any number of characters to be sent starting at the nominated position; with an output from the computer a sufficient number of characters will cause wrapping back to the start of the screen, and even overwriting of the early part of

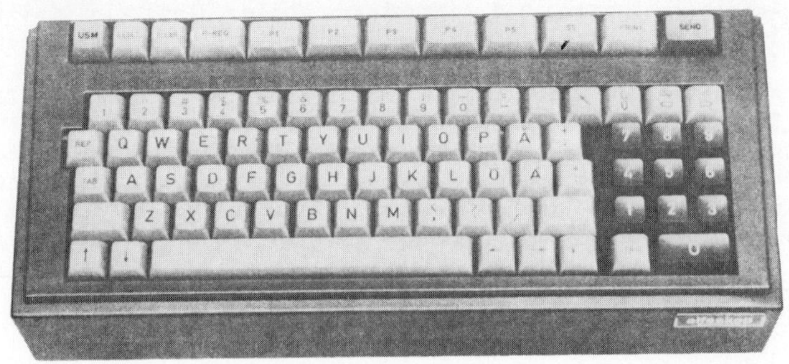

FIG 5-2 KEYBOARD OF ALFASCOPE TERMINAL

the same message. The keyboard is locked during transmission of any message, and while transmission is pending.

At the completion of an output message the cursor is routinely in the next screen location; however, it can be relocated by the computer as part of the one transmission before the keyboard is unlocked again.

The characters transmitted in a message from the terminal are demarcated as to their end by the cursor, and as to their beginning by the last start-of-message character (the graphic '┏') preceding it, or, failing such a character, the home position. All such messages explicitly start at the starting position. The SEND key at the top right of the keyboard must be pressed to cause transmission from the terminal.

Besides this ability to delimit a sub-section of the screen, the terminal has a tab feature and the communications logic suppresses trailing spaces in each row.

The Alfascope - System conventions and practices

Of the 16 rows available for data on the Alfascope screen, only the upper 14 are used for keyboard entry in the Stockholm System. Though obviously tightening one constraint, this arrangement allows a general latitude for a computer response without disturbing the user's entry. While a total or near-total alteration of screen contents must necessarily occur very often, the System has, as a design principle, commonly the repetition to the user of his message, augmented by directions, advice or other response. In responding to a query for information, the computer can, of course, use these later lines just as the earlier ones for its display of the information.

Standard conventions apply also to the first three lines of the screen, the first being used for the basic code and identification details concerning the current activity, the second for a textual interpretation of that code, and the third for instructions about answering then, in turn, the answer.

As illustrated below and detailed in succeeding chapters, using the

System involves the alternating transmission of two or more messages between terminal (user) and computer. While the initiative rests essentially with the user, control rests essentially with the computer. The set of messages concerning any one independent piece of business - be it an enquiry, an admission, a booking or set of bookings, etc., is called here a dialog. Such a dialog as a simple enquiry reaches its conclusion with the initial computer response, which then states the fact in the bottom row of the screen. Other dialogs proceed through many messages, and through one or more points at which the user must make some choice. Indeed, until the dialog is concluded, the user always has the choice of continuing or breaking the dialog, but on occasions there is a choice of alternative routes of continuation or a choice of data alternatives (e.g. of visit or of appointment).

Row 3 routinely enunciates the alternatives available, and provides space at its right-hand-end, in the last 16 positions, for the answer, being typically a standard short word or a line-identifying number. Where a dialog is to cause the updating of any file, the penultimate step is the checking by computer of the whole and direction, if satisfactory, of the user to register the transaction or break (i.e. abort) the dialog.

Until 1975, all such user answers, plus the user action to close a terminal session (and thereby close the opening effected by initial submission and acceptance of a security password), were effected by this procedure involving keying of an answer into the screen. Though the main answers were in fact acceptable as only two letters, the function keys offered more efficient means for such frequent actions. Now, four of the most common actions are executable by use of these keys, namely

Function key 1 Break dialog ('BREAK')
Function key 2 Turn to next page ('NEXT_PAGE')
Function key 3 Turn to preceding page ('BACK')
Function key 4 Register transaction(s) ('REG')

(The non-use of the fifth function key of the Alfascope is caused by the Uniscopes having only four such keys.)

The first of these is shown on many of the illustrative screen displays below as 'BREAK' or 'BREAK DIALOG', and will be referred to as 'break' etc., in the text. The last is shown in illustrations as 'REG' and the process referred to in the text as registering of data. Reference to such actions, or to the general process of 'answering', will be taken as inferring the transmission of the message involved.

The positions 48 through 64 on row 3, generally reserved for the answer that is keyed to the screen, is referred to as the 'answer zone', unless explicit qualification is applied to that expression. Where a screen entry is required or expected of the user, the cursor is automatically placed by the computer at position 49, with a start-of-message symbol in position 48 so as to simplify the user's task. Hence, the mere keying of the answering character or characters, plus depression of the SEND key, is all that is required of the user.

USING A TERMINAL

Activating a terminal

Having switched on the terminal and allowed it some 30 seconds to warm up, a user must first reposition the cursor to the home position. Then, to initiate a session the user must enter

SP nnnnn

where nnnnn represents the user's external security code (the significance of which is discussed in Chapter 12).

The initial characters SP are the code for this session-initiating dialog, and like all such codes represents a meaningful abbreviation of the name of the dialog - in this case 'sekretess pa' or 'secrecy on'. (Except for avoiding the unique Scandinavian letters, the Swedish dialog code values are retained in this text, but the dialog name is rendered in English. This tends to obscure the relationship between the two, but should be borne in mind when reading the descriptions below.) The dialog codes range up to five characters in length.

If the entered security code is not acceptable, notice of rejection appears on the screen below the user's entry. The user can repeat the initial process following a first failure, and repeated up to a limit currently set at four failures, after which the computer closes the terminal.

Acceptance of an entered security code is signified by a response that states the date and time that the code was last accepted.

Having been accepted by the System, the user is now free to proceed to any transactional dialog within the established repertoire. These vary from a complicated booking dialog that may involve a dozen or more messages being transmitted each way to a simple query-then-response dialog that is ended by the first computer response. The latter example has no impact on the files, while others may involve changes to several different records in different files. (This much-varying entity is called a 'transaktion' in Swedish but with such characteristics it seems more conveniently called a dialog.)

The additional functions of retrieving H.R. information and searching for PERSON-NUMB that are included in Fig 5-1 are each covered by one dialog, with codes HRO and PNR respectively. Both are without effect on the records, but are good examples of the accessing of the data base via a terminal.

Dialog PNR, PERSON-NUMB search

The facility to search for a PERSON-NUMB has already been referred to in the discussion of the H.R. in Chapter 4. A PNR search can be initiated by transmission of the mere message

PNR

located, as usual, at the top left of the screen. In response the computer states the variables that can be entered, plus a couple of illustrative examples; Fig 5-3 shows this response (translated, as are all subsequent screen displays, into English in a manner that retains the Swedish format and style).

```
-----------------------------------------------------------------------
--                                                                   --
-- PNR                                                               --
-- PERSON-NUMB SEARCH                                                --
-- GIVE ONE OR MORE OF FOLLOWING FACTS                               --
--                                                                   --
--   SURNAME         (FIRST FIVE LETTERS)                            --
--   SEX             (M OR F)                                        --
--   BIRTH-YEAR      (FIXED YEAR OR INTERVAL)                        --
--   BIRTH-MONTH                                                     --
--   BIRTH-DAY                                                       --
--                                                                   --
-- EXAMPLES:                                                         --
-- PNR  PALME  M  1920-30                                            --
-- PNR  BERGH  K  1869 11 27                                         --
--                                                                   --
-- DIALOG CLOSED                                                     --
--                                                                   --
--                                                                   --
-----------------------------------------------------------------------
```

FIG 5-3 PNR - INITIAL RESPONSE WHEN NO NUMBER ENTERED

Of the indicated data, only the surname component is obligatory. However, if any one of the other four is not entered, all subsequent ones must be omitted. As stated, only the first five letters of the surname are entered - the extra letters having been deemed of insufficient weight to warrant storage in the indexing file (Name file) used. The sex question can be explicitly answered with X if unknown. If the precise birthyear is not known, a range such as 1920-30 can be shown, as per the first-displayed example.

However, while apparently seeking data from the user, this response from the computer has, as stated in its last displayed line, closed the initiated dialog. At this juncture, the user could, without further ado, proceed to some different dialog. However, presuming a desire to pursue the identification of a person, the appropriate step now - and one that could have been made at the outset - is to enter and transmit PNR and the indicated information, in the manner illustrated by examples in Fig 5-3, e.g.

PNR PETTE M 1929 02 08

or

PNR KARLS X 1912-20

or

PNR JOHAN

This one line of information is placed at the top of the screen. If following a preceding PNR dialog, entry can be done by movement of the cursor to the second position after the already displayed PNR dialog code, then entry of the identification data. At no time in such a situation does the screen need to be cleared before or after keyboard entry; it suffices to have the first line correct up to the cursor position, then press the SEND key. At such a juncture the computer receives and peruses only the limited data zone applicable, because of the part-screen transmission scheme described earlier.

The System response to this search message is a list of all persons meeting the stated criteria, giving for each the full name and address, plus occupation/title, alongside the full PERSON-NUMB. Fig 5-4 illustrates

```
--------------------------------------------------------------------------------
--                                                                            --
-- PNR LINDB M 1929 02 08                                                     --
-- PERSON-NUMB SEARCH                                                         --
--                                                                            --
-- 1  290208-0890  LINDBORG, KURT EMANUEL        DIRECTOR                     --
--                 #2-144 MOUNTAIN ST      11231 STOCKHOLM                    --
-- 2  290208-0114  LINDBERG, SVEN EFRAIM         MECHANIC                     --
--                 #2-26 HILLVIEW AV       11727 NYNASHAMN                    --
--                                                                            --
--                                                                            --
--                                                                            --
--                                                                            --
--                                                                            --
--                                                                            --
--                                                                            --
--                                                                            --
--                                                                            --
--                                                                            --
--------------------------------------------------------------------------------
```

FIG 5-4 PNR - INITIAL RESPONSE TO ENTERED NUMBER

a more conservative response with only two persons meeting the criteria. The screen can accommodate at most six persons in such manner; the occurrence of further persons is signified by CONTD displayed at the bottom right of the screen. The next batch of persons can be seen by pressing the NEXT PAGE key, this procedure being repeatable as appropriate. Pressing of the BACK key then the SEND key reverses this process.

If this display provides the information required, the dialog can be terminated by the standard procedure of pressing the BREAK key. Such action is necessary even if another PNR dialog is required, either for another person or, using different data, the same person. The latter situation can arise where the pertinent person does not show in the list and, for instance, some alternative spelling of name may be appropriate, or where the displayed list is unmanageably long and some additional constriction is warranted. Regarding the name, it must be appreciated that the manner of updating the H.R. favors a lower error-rate than would be true for most hospital records, so that care with the spelling of the current patient's name should be effective regarding name matching. However, not only are there naturally some errors, but foreign names can present problems if they contain letters outside of the Swedish alphabet or other reason for varying the original spelling. There is no automatic simplification - phonetic or other - carried out, so any alternatives must be explicitly pursued by the user. The user manual says "a little imagination is sometimes needed".

If further information is required on a person included in the list, this can be obtained to a limited extent by the user indicating the individual and entering one of the alternatives HRU, CFU, KRM, RTG or SLV to indicate the need for different types of information. Each of these is a distinct dialog in itself, discussed below, and their entry at this juncture effectively terminates the PNR dialog and simultaneously opens the new one.

Indication of the relevant person in the list is made using the line number already explicitly displayed on the screen. (Note that, though being the figures 1, 2, ..., they occur on the 4th, 6th, ... of the 14 rows provide by the c.r.t. screen. The term 'row' is herein used in this latter sense and the term 'line', as pertaining to a screen, used for the logical entity exemplified in Fig 5-4.) This is followed by the chosen dialog code in the manner,

2 KRM,

this composite entry being made in the standard answer zone of the screen. Routine pressing of the SEND key conveys the answer to the computer.

Dialogs HRO; CFU; KRM; RTG; SLV - information retrieval from H.R.

Each of these five dialog codes provides the means to access a distinct subset of the information recorded in H.R. for a person, the subsets being

HRO an overview of the facility
CFU the central registry information
KRM the critical medical information
RTG the X-ray records
SLV the inpatient records.

Initiation of any one of the five is fundamentally the same, being transmission of the dialog code plus identification of the patient. Neglecting indirect entry as from the PNR dialog, this means entering the chosen code then the pertinent PERSON-NUMB in row 1 and transmitting, eg.

KRM 000101-0073

The responses are exemplified respectively in Figs. 5-5 thru 5-9. In these it can be seen that the original opening line has been augmented by the name of the patient, and the second row of the screen, in a manner already shown with PNR and standard for the System, provides the full title

```
HRO 000101+0073            JACOBSON, PETER JAMES
HUVUD REGISTER OVERVIEW

CFU  CENTRAL CENSUS REGISTRY DATA
KRM  CRITICAL MEDICAL DATA
RTG  X-RAY DATA
SLV  INPATIENT DATA
```

FIG 5-5 HRO - INITIAL RESPONSE

that the dialog code represents.

As Fig 5-5 shows, beyond the name for the given PERSON-NUMB, the HRO provides no information from H.R. but merely a list of the other dialogs.

```
¬¬¬¬¬¬¬¬¬¬¬¬¬¬¬¬¬¬¬¬¬¬¬¬¬¬¬¬¬¬¬¬¬¬¬¬¬¬¬¬¬¬¬¬¬¬¬¬¬¬¬¬¬¬¬¬¬¬¬¬¬¬¬¬¬¬¬¬¬¬
¬¬                                                                  ¬¬
¬¬ CFU 000101+0073              JACOBSON, PETER JAMES               ¬¬
¬¬ CENTRAL CENSUS REGISTRY DATA                                     ¬¬
¬¬                                                                  ¬¬
¬¬ STREET ADDRESS 8 THE STRAND                                      ¬¬
¬¬                11977 STOCKHOLM                                   ¬¬
¬¬                                                                  ¬¬
¬¬ MUNICIPALITY 80 BROMMA       PARISH 16  TRACT 46                 ¬¬
¬¬ CENSUS YR          1920                                          ¬¬
¬¬                                                                  ¬¬
¬¬ CITIZENSHIP  SWEDISH                                             ¬¬
¬¬ OCCP         TIMBERMAN                  PENSIONED 1950           ¬¬
¬¬ CIVIL STATUS MARRIED      170202        ASSOC NR 000202+0063     ¬¬
¬¬                                                                  ¬¬
¬¬                                                                  ¬¬
¬¬                                                                  ¬¬
¬¬                                                                  ¬¬
¬¬                                                                  ¬¬
¬¬¬¬¬¬¬¬¬¬¬¬¬¬¬¬¬¬¬¬¬¬¬¬¬¬¬¬¬¬¬¬¬¬¬¬¬¬¬¬¬¬¬¬¬¬¬¬¬¬¬¬¬¬¬¬¬¬¬¬¬¬¬¬¬¬¬¬¬¬
```

FIG 5-6 CFU - INITIAL RESPONSE

```
¬¬¬¬¬¬¬¬¬¬¬¬¬¬¬¬¬¬¬¬¬¬¬¬¬¬¬¬¬¬¬¬¬¬¬¬¬¬¬¬¬¬¬¬¬¬¬¬¬¬¬¬¬¬¬¬¬¬¬¬¬¬¬¬¬¬¬¬¬¬
¬¬                                                                  ¬¬
¬¬ KRM 000101+0073              JACOBSON, PETER JAMES               ¬¬
¬¬ CRITICAL MEDICAL DATA                                            ¬¬
¬¬                                                                  ¬¬
¬¬ TELEFON     HOME       08/616263      WORK                       ¬¬
¬¬                                                                  ¬¬
¬¬ BLOODGROUP  AB+    1 GROUPING                                    ¬¬
¬¬ CRIT DISEASES                                                    ¬¬
¬¬ VACC                                                             ¬¬
¬¬                                                                  ¬¬
¬¬                                                                  ¬¬
¬¬                                                                  ¬¬
¬¬                                                                  ¬¬
¬¬                                                                  ¬¬
¬¬                                                                  ¬¬
¬¬                                                                  ¬¬
¬¬                                                                  ¬¬
¬¬                                                                  ¬¬
¬¬¬¬¬¬¬¬¬¬¬¬¬¬¬¬¬¬¬¬¬¬¬¬¬¬¬¬¬¬¬¬¬¬¬¬¬¬¬¬¬¬¬¬¬¬¬¬¬¬¬¬¬¬¬¬¬¬¬¬¬¬¬¬¬¬¬¬¬¬
```

FIG 5-7 KRM - INITIAL RESPONSE

While this is the most efficient means of obtaining only the name, the main purpose of this dialog, like the PNR dialog without any personal data, is to provide a lead-off for the less familiar user.

Of the other four, CFU provides a standard screen of data and KRM could only exceed a screenful in highly exceptional circumstance; in contrast, RTG and SLV both seek information that can readily exceed the amount intelligibly displayed at one moment. Since only 10 rows are available for the display of successive visits, even with each visit occupying one row, it is quite conceivable for the response to an RTG or even an SLV to exceed one screenful. Further, the total information available per inpatient stay can not be displayed in one row, while that

```
--------------------------------------------------------------------------
--                                                                      --
-- RTG 000101+0073                    JACOBSON, PETER JAMES             --
-- EARLIER X-RAY EXAMINATIONS                                           --
--                                                                      --
--    1 DS    URO   401124            530                               --
--    2 DS    SUR   400622            510                               --
--    3 DS    SUR   400525            453                               --
--    4 DS    SUR   400525            320                               --
--    5 DS    SUR   400522            420                               --
--    6 DS    SUR   400520            510                               --
--    7 DS    MED   370418            320                               --
--                                                                      --
--                                                                      --
--                                                                      --
--                                                                      --
--                                                                      --
--                                                                      --
--                                                                      --
--------------------------------------------------------------------------
```

<u>FIG</u> 5-8 RTG - INITIAL RESPONSE (OVERVIEW)

```
--------------------------------------------------------------------------
--                                                                      --
-- SLV 000101+0073                    JACOBSON, PETER JAMES             --
-- EARLIER ADMISSIONS                                                   --
--                                                                      --
--    1  DS  URO  410331    61200*                                      --
--    2  DS  SUR  400513    60218    58499*                             --
--                                                                      --
--                                                                      --
--                                                                      --
--                                                                      --
--                                                                      --
--                                                                      --
--                                                                      --
--                                                                      --
--                                                                      --
--                                                                      --
--    * DIAGNOSIS THAT REQUIRED OPERATION                               --
--                                                                      --
--------------------------------------------------------------------------
```

<u>FIG</u> 5-9 SLV - INITIAL RESPONSE (OVERVIEW)

for the RTG could only be so done if full coding is adopted, and intelligibility is regarded as requiring textual interpretation of diagnoses for instance.

The summary information shown for each x-ray is, successively, line number within list, institution, requisitioning department and body part. For each inpatient stay it is similar up to the date, which is that of admission, then comes diagnoses. Any continuation of lists beyond a single screen is indicated and dealt with in the manner already described for PNR. For RTG and SLV, the brief information shown in the listings can be expanded upon by entry of the appropriate line number in the answer zone - being the position of cursor set by the computer message. Transmission of this number brings, for the indicated x-ray or inpatient stay, the detailed display of Fig 5-10 or 5-11 respectively. It should be noted that, for obvious convenience, these lists start with the most recent and proceed in reverse chronology. These detailed displays, like those for CFU and KRM, are largely self-explanatory regarding their contents.

```
RTG 000101+0073            JACOBSON, PETER JAMES
EARLIER X-RAY EXAMINATIONS

 3 DS   SUR            400525

   ORGAN    453    CHOLIANGIOGRAM

   METHOD     7    DYEING

   FINDING   14
```

FIG 5-10 RTG - DETAILED RESPONSE

```
SLV 000101+0073            JACOBSON, PETER JAMES
EARLIER ADMISSIONS

 2 DS   SUR  400513/HOME  -400529/HOME          EMERGENCY

DIAGNOSIS    60218  URETHRAL CALCULUS
DIAGNOSIS    58499  CHOLELITHIASIS
OPN           5350  CHOLECYSTECTOMY
OPN             57  CHOLIANGIOGRAM DURING OP





    ( ) WITHIN PARENTHESES IS ENTERED ANESTHESIA CODE AND
RNR USED AT ADMISSION.
```

FIG 5-11 SLV - DETAILED RESPONSE

With the display of such details the cursor is left in the normal answer zone, and entry of a number plus depression of the SEND key will repeat the detailing process for the indicated line. Alternatively, transmission of the current dialog code as answer will re-establish the patient list, and transmission of one of the related codes will change the dialog while maintaining the same patient as the subject. When all information of interest has been retrieved, depression of the BREAK key closes the current dialog and drops the subject patient.

Obtaining a local printout

The usual equipment provisions of the County include a slave printer with each single or small cluster of normal terminals. These, as mentioned, are able to print from the control memory that is used for refreshing the c.r.t. display. In the case of a cluster, facility exists for one printer to print from any of the memory sections for up to four terminals.

Obtaining a print-out on a slave printer, assuming the device is 'on', is simply a matter of pressing the PRINT key. During the print-out, plus any preceding wait for a shared printer, the keyboard is locked. The characters printed are the same as those that would have been transmitted had the SEND key been depressed, and not necessarily the whole screen. Hence there may be a need to insert or remove a start-of-message character and to re-position the cursor before the PRINT key is pressed. The layout of the printed characters is essentially that of them on the screen, except that the tab character does not occupy the character position that it does on the screen.

An incoming message from the computer can be directed automatically to the printer as well as the screen. (A facility also exists, via the P-REQ key, for the user to have the computer take the message and send it back to the printer - so as to avoid immediate delay of other work or because of a temporary printer problem, but this is not currently implemented.) The existence of the pending return transmission, like that of any message initiated by the computer and awaiting opportunity for display, is indicated on the terminal by illumination of the USM key. Depression of this key at a convenient time brings transmission. By chaining output messages, the computer can send a communication of over 1024 characters to the printer.

Dialog RNR - obtaining a RESV-NUMBER

The need for RESV-NUMBER (or RNR) in place of the normal PERSON-NUMB (or PNR) was discussed in Chapter 4 in the context of the P.R. Since obtaining an RNR value is the one remaining significant dialog that is separate from any one application, it is appropriate to describe it here as a further example of using a terminal.

Opening this dialog involves only the message

RNR s

where s = M for male, F for female. The computer response, beyond the addition of the dialog name in row 2, is merely the display of the newly assigned number plus the full phrase for sex, followed by the statement that the number has now been assigned.

The RNR, it will be recollected, begins with two digits representing institution. Though no reference is made to the institution in the requesting message, the institution of the user is always known from the security code submitted in the dialog that opened the terminal session, and the institutional location of each terminal is also known to the computer.

The computer uses the latter in the case of assigning an RNR.

APPLICATION PROGRAMS

As is to be expected, the application programs have been designed as a set of modules to be called individually as message traffic demands. Any one dialog involves an unbounded chain of programs. The typical chain involves up to five programs, and fits into one common style, viz

- first - an initialized program, which establishes the intial conditions pertinent to the dialog, then
- second - a display program, which puts out the various requests and responses that the dialog prompts, then
- third - a validation program, which carries out all the specified validatory checks for the user's response to a display, then (unless failure requires a return to the second program)
- fourth - an update program, which effects any updating arising, then
- fifth - a close-out program.

At the completion of any one program, control is surrendered to the MIDAS system using the command CALL or LINK, together with identification of the program to be called next for the task at hand. Control is also surrendered to the operating system whenever an input/output operation is initiated on a temporary basis for the program concerned (using the standard operating system feature).

Some of the dialogs already illustrated only seek information; they have no power to alter the data base and hence no need for an update program in their chain. However, while the provision of such 'see-only' dialogs is widespread in the System, virtually all are directly associated with an update dialog. Yet further, they are indeed associated usually with two update dialogs - one that creates a record (e.g. of a booking, an admission, etc.) and one that amends such a record. Since these three dialogs - the create, the amend, and the 'see-only' - have considerable procedures and literal values in common for any one record-type, it is usual to service them by one common chain. Where appropriate the update is omitted (which, of course, can happen both through non-completion of an updating dialog and, more positively, a decision not to amend after the existing record has been displayed as well as through choice of a non-updating dialog). However, except for this omission - and still greater omission if the dialog is aborted by lack of user response to a display call, the procedures for all three routes are called in as one program at each step in the chain, rather than called selectively as sub-modules.

The size of the modules vary considerably. As illustration, the one chain serving the dialogs that relate to patients being on the waiting list (actually 5 programs in total) have the following dimensions

- Initialize program - 1120 words from 278 MIDAS statements
- Display program - 540 words from 124 MIDAS statements
- Validation program - 1712 words from 269 MIDAS statements
- Update program - 520 words from 47 MIDAS statements
- Close-out program - 40 words from 13 MIDAS statements

where the storage requirements pertain to main (core) store and include both program and data. The waiting list application involves three separate chains, but with a common close-out program, - hence 13 programs.

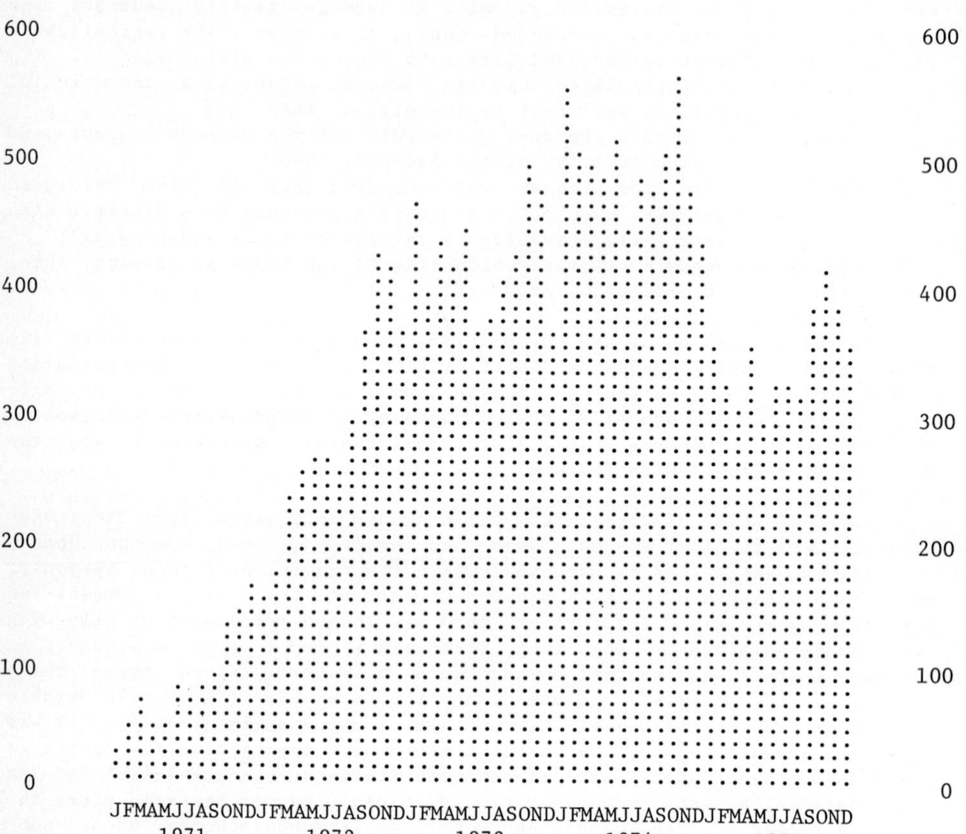

FIG 5-12 DIALOGS PER MONTH, 1971-1975

NOTE: THE STATISTICS FOR 1975 EXCLUDE A TYPE OF INTERNAL DIALOG THAT ROUGHLY DOUBLED THE FIGURES FOR PRECEDING YEARS.

Despite the considerable consolidation of the routines, the number of program-load calls is seen as one of the critical factors for processing capacity. One factor exacerbating this problem is the omission from MIDAS of a composite facility for surrendering control because of an input instruction and simultaneously establishing the recall to a different program. Pending provision of such a facility, the display program is routinely recalled just for it to call the validation program.

THE ACTIVITY LOAD

The number of dialogs per month has risen from about 30 000 at the beginning of 1971 to around 500 000 through most of 1974. Because of changes in definitions plus introduction of some multi-transaction dialog types, particular referable to laboratories, the number of dialogs averaged about only 350 0000 per month during 1976, as Fig. 5-12 shows. Another factor influencing this variability, more especially gross month-to-month variation, has been the spasmodic load of conversions; as each additional hospital was brought within any application, there was necessarily a conspicuous one-time traffic load.

The load incurred by the hardware, software and communication lines is indicated by Table 5-l and associated tables in the succeeding five chapters. As Table 5-1 shows, the average dialog involves five messages one way or the other along a line, adding up to nearly 1000 characters being transmitted. At the computer, this average dialog necessitates 24 accesses to disc or tape, with 11 000 words being transferred thereby, and seven program calls; total central processor time required is 0.39 secs including input/putput handling.

That average overall picture is far from representative of even the average within particular applications. In most regards the chemical laboratory application averages about five times the overall average. The main counterbalance comes from the general enquiry dialogs discussed above, and similar enquiry dialogs available to the housing authority.

The average number of program calls, which for the waiting list is shown as just equal to the number of programs in the processing chain, is elevated in some other applications by options to chain transactions, to process multiple transactions or to be repetitious (e.g. in pursuit of a suitable booking time).

The contents of Table 5-1 derive from a study conducted during 1 thru 5 September 1975, - a period free of any gross special effects and so reasonably representative of 'normal business', although seen as somewhat understating the load because of the lingering affect of summer vacations. Those were weekdays; week-end traffic is significant but very much less. Concurrent observations of the telecommunication lines indicated that no line was loaded to more than 50% of its capacity over any period of 15 minutes.

DIALOG	AVERAGE IMPACT PER DIALOG						DAILY TRAFFIC		
	TELECOMS		OTHER I/O		PROG	CPU			
	MSGS	CHARS	ACC	KWDS	CALLS	SECS	MIN	MEAN	MAX
SP	2	123	6	-	1	.04	1354	1632	1823
PNR	4	831	14	9	2	.20	1565	1856	2191
SLV	3	342	10	8	1	.32	89	215	49
WTGL	5	1770	14	10	5	.33	1311	1530	1888
INPAT	4	1081	17	9	9	.26	2515	2922	3194
BOOK	5	1400	58	22	12	.94	644	852	1145
OUTP	4	1116	14	11	4	.28	748	868	1108
CHEM	8	2250	119	51	33	1.90	1297	1636	1844
HOUSG	5	812	13	8	2	.20	1272	1651	1918
ETC									
OVERALL	5	955	24	11	7	.39	14226	16008	17704

TABLE 5-1 REAL-TIME PROCESSING STATISTICS FOR SYSTEM, BASED ON SURVEY OF 1 THRU 5 SEP 75.

AVERAGE IMPACT PER DIALOG SHOWS NUMBER OF 1-WAY MESSAGES AND NUMBER OF DATA CHARACTERS TRANSMITTED OVER TELECOMMUNICATION LINES; NUMBER OF READ OR WRITE ACCESSES TO DISKS AND LOG TAPE, PLUS NUMBER OF THOUSANDS OF WORDS TRANSFERRED; NUMBER OF PROGRAM MODULES CALLED AND THE SECONDS OF C.P.U. EXECUTION TIME.

DAILY TRAFFIC SHOWS THE NUMBER OF DIALOGS PER DAY, IN TERMS OF THE MINIMUM, THE MEAN, AND THE MAXIMUM; OVER THE FIVE CONSECUTIVE WEEKDAYS INCLUDED IN THE SURVEY.

WTG L, INPAT,.. CHEM REPRESENT THE OVERALL PICTURE FOR THE FIVE SUB-SYSTEMS DISCUSSED.

HOUSG REPRESENTS THE OVERALL PICTURE FOR THE HOUSING DEPT. APPLICATIONS.

'ETC' COVERS MISCELLANEOUS DIALOGS NOT INCLUDED ABOVE.

CHAPTER 6

WAITING LIST SUB-SYSTEM

As outlined in Chapter 2, the waiting list application maintains an inventory of unmet demand, and has been implemented across the whole County on an integrated basis. It applies equally to outpatient as to inpatient services, but does not cover such things as general appointments with doctors as distinct from specific investigatory or therapeutic procedures.

Besides the direct use as a queue for patients and a pool of customers to be assigned the existing facilities as they have vacancies, impending or actual, the waiting list is also seen as of significant value for the proper advance planning of a patient's visit and for the planning of the provision and operation of facilities. Thus it has been designed to include, beside the identity of each waiting patient and the primary service required, information on urgency, accommodation preferences, estimated length of stay and/or additional services required. (The Swedish name for the sub-system is literally "care planning", though it has always been rendered "waiting list" in English publications.)

RECORDING THE NEED

Such wider information generally requires the attention of additional consultative staff to the physician making the basic request for a service. While this consultation could be made following a rudimentary entry of the patient's data to the computerized waiting list, and the supplementary information added as a subsequent update, the procedure established is based on initial entry of the total picture on a paper form, then entry to the computer, usually via the batch data route. The haste of immediate computer processing is rarely needed; where haste is required, outside of the normal emergency department proceedings, it is more a matter of having the consultative assessment made promptly than having to have real-time input. And, even for non-emergency-department cases, manual override of computerized waiting list and bookings can always be effected.

The basic step

The basic document is then a form, and this is displayed, in its Swedish, in Fig 6-1.

Following the typical identification and contact information, plus record of referring doctor and place (notes 1 thru 7 in figure), the form provides space for diagnoses then services demanded. In this example of diabetes mellitus, no operations or special investigatory tests are shown as needed other than the standard tests upon admission. The last - under note 9 - can be omitted and non-standard tests at admission can be specified in the free text area (to 39 characters). Above, up to three post-admission procedures can be specified, each with its own stated delay after admission, plus code and name of procedure, then name and code of specific doctor involved. Each procedure involved may be an operation, an investigatory test, an examination, or a therapeutic procedure.

Vårdinrättning (anges endast om denna ej framgår av vidstående ruta)

Vårdplan

☐ Ändring/komplettering*

Personnr 000101+0073

Namn Peterson, Peter James ❶

Gatuadress Strandvägen 8

Postadress inkl postnr 119 77 STOCKHOLM

Telefon 08/61 62 63 ❷

Ev vårdnadshavare

Datum 750820 ❸

11002 Inrättning nr | 101 Klinik nr | Subspec/avd

Vårdplanen är uppgjord av (namn och tjänsteställe)

L. Lj. ❹

Kompletterande uppgifter om patienten

X Man ☐ Kvinna | Sysselsättning Timmerman | Nat om ej svensk

Inremitterande instans (läkare)

Inremitterande instans (läkare). Om inrättnkod saknas skall inrättningens- eller läkarens namn och adress anges med högst 20 tecken

❺ Dr. Test med. mott.

Inrättning nr | Klinik nr | Vårdtyp Ö ❻

Kallelse adress

X hemmet (se ovan) ☐ Inremitterande instans (läkare) ❼

Diagnos

Diagnoskod | Diagnos i klartext (15 tecken per rad)

Diabetes mellitus ❽

Resurskrävande undersökningar/operationer

Antal dagar efter intagningen	Kod (4 tecken)	Undersökningar/operationer etc	Läkare	Läkarkod (4 tecken)

Önskade undersökningar i samband med intagningen ❾

X Standard-prov | Övrigt (fri text om högst 39 tecken)

Intagning (prioritet, kritiskt datum, vårdtid, etc)

patienten är ❿ ☐ Infekterad | ☐ FF dubbel förtur | X F enkel förtur ⓫ | ☐ N normal förtur 1 | ☐ I normal förtur 2 | ☐ P platsbokad | rumtyp X fler-bädd | ☐ 2 bädd ⓬ | ☐ 1 bädd

Inplaneringskod (2 tecken) ⓭ | Planerad intagningsdatum (år, mån, dag) ⓮ | Kritiskt datum (år, mån, dag) ⓯ | Förväntad vårdtid (antal dagar 2 tecken) | Vårdtyngd (patientklass, 2 tecken)

Anmärkningar samt patientens önskemål om intagning (20 tecken per rad)

⓰ Sjukskr. fr.o.m. 17.8 -75

2 d varsel

Beslut om intagning

Beslutsdatum	Intagningsdatum	Kontaktdatum	Avdelning	Resultat av förfrågan		
				☐ patient och sjukhus har godkänt intagningsdatum	☐ patienten avböjt	☐ sjukhuset avböjt
				☐ patient och sjukhus har godkänt intagningsdatum	☐ patienten avböjt	☐ sjukhuset avböjt
				☐ patient och sjukhus har godkänt intagningsdatum	☐ patienten avböjt	☐ sjukhuset avböjt

Patienten avregistrerad från vårdplan datum ☐ intagen ☐ akut ☐ avliden ☐ fel. registrering ☐ övrigt ⓱

* Vid ändring eller komplettering skall endast personnummer, namn samt ändrade data ifyllas

B 1371-02A

FIG 6-1 REGISTRATION FORM FOR WAITING LIST.

A place to denote an infectious patient (note 10) is followed by an array of priority alternatives (note 11) in accordance with standards of the County Social Welfare Department, described in Chapter 2, but augmented by

I meaning very low priority (i.e. unnecessary)
P meaning that a place has been booked.

The value I has been added to deal with such situations as very old people having small benign tumors that would more generally be regarded as in need of excision. The value P indicates the scope for by-passing the delay in processing the form.

The room-type (note 12) is merely an expression of patient's preference, while note 13 indicates scope for a local code that can be used for sorting or selecting waiting-list patients in accord with particular requirements of the consulted department. Notes 14 and 15 identify fields used for more urgent cases, the first accommodating the date for admission if already established, the second the critical date for admission. Use of the latter is well illustrated by abortions, but it applies to many other procedures and situations. The succeeding fields are for expected length of stay and the code for loading class, i.e. the relative load on nursing care of the patient, which depends both on the procedures required and the physical condition of the patient.

Space for free-text remarks of special patient needs, related care, and so on (note 16), is followed by an area for manual recording of booking and admission, the last line of which (note 17) is subsequently used for updating the waiting list by removal of the listed patient.

<u>Dialogs VPL/VPLO - registering a patient in the waiting list</u>

The dialogs VPL and VPLO provide for registering a patient in the waiting list, respectively for inpatient and for outpatient service.

Transmission of the dialog code plus <u>P</u>N<u>R</u>/<u>R</u>N<u>R</u> results in display on the screen of a form completed to the extent possible from the H.R. for patients included therein. Fig 6-2 illustrates a response for the case of Fig 6-1, assuming that the patient is in the H.R. It is not necessary that the fields common to the paper form and the H.R. have the same values; not only might the patient have given a new or forthcoming address, for instance, but the telephone number is only updated through contact with the health services and could be years out of date.

The operator must complete appropriate vacant fields in the form display and alter those that differ from the paper form, then transmit the completed form (ensuring that the cursor is beyond the last field). Three of the fields - ADAT being date of any subsequent amendment and the last two, which record the date and reason for ultimate removal from the waiting list - are inherently unusable at this juncture.

In the standard practice of the System, the entered data is at this point only inspected by the computer, bringing in row 3 a statement on its acceptability and, if errors occur, blinking characters alongside each end of each aberrant field. If the data is acceptable the process is completed by pressing of the REG key then transmission; if unacceptable appropriate amendment must be made and the form re-submitted by pressing the TRANSMIT key. In either case there is the alternative of discontinuing the dialog by

```
-----------------------------------------------------------------------------
--                                                                         --
-- VPL   000101+0073                                                       --
-- WAITING LIST                                                            --
-- ENTER NEW DATA OR BREAK                          r                    r --
--  PNR   000101+0073                               SEX M                  --
--  NAME PETERSON, PETER JAMES............... OCCP TIMBERMAN               --
--  ADDR 8 THE STRAND.............. PONR 11977 PT STOCKHOLM                --
--  TEL  123456.....    TEL ...........                  INF N             --
--  RDAT 750611   ADAT ......  INSTN .....  DEPT ....  STN ...             --
--  REF DOC ....................                                           --
--  DIAGNOS ..............  CD .....  NOTE ..................              --
--  DIAGNOS ..............  CD .....  NOTE ..................              --
--  DIAGNOS ..............  CD .....  NOTE ..................              --
--  PRTY N. ACC S PATNTC .. PLDATE ......  CRITDATE ......                 --
--  OPDAY ..  OPNC ....    REMDATE ......  REMCD .......                   --
--                                                                         --
--                                                                         --
--                                                                         --
-----------------------------------------------------------------------------
```

FIG 6-2 VPL & VPLO - INITIAL RESPONSE

pressing the BREAK key and transmitting.

Dialog VPLK - alter a registration in the waiting list

Transmission of the dialog code VPLK plus PNR/RNR is the first step toward altering (including cancelling) a registration in the waiting list. The immediate response to this merely seeks the answer as to whether it is an inpatient or an outpatient case, to which the operator must respond in the normal answering manner.

If the patient has multiple registrations in the indicated category, the next response lists them in chronological order of insertion, with numbered lines containing brief status information besides the date of registration. Entry of the pertinent line number in row 3 and transmission brings the computer to the particular registration concerned, displayed in the same layout as with VPL, VPLO.

The recording via VPLK that a patient has been provided with the demanded service, or at least admitted to hospital for the purpose, does not in itself remove the record from the waiting list. This happens after; in the meantime the record remains as visible as others, its cancellation date showing the difference.

Dialog VPLU - obtaining information from waiting list

The VPLU dialog functions similarly to VPLK but has no capability for altering the recorded information. Since display of the required information achieves the objective of VPLU, the computer closes the dialog with the display.

PLANNING THE PROVISION OF SERVICE

Planning the admission or other servicing of patients in the waiting list requires, cf course, access to the aggregate record of demand, i.e. sight of the waiting list in some selective sense. Currently the total waiting list in the County exceeds 30 000 people, and even the sub-list for some individual types of service is very long.

Although the associated file is integrated over the whole County, each recorded demand is associated with a particular facility through the consultative stage passed before entry to the computer. Institution and department are recorded, the latter being often a sub-specialty rather than specialty.

To allow each department to deal with its unmet demand, various reports are available from Datacentral, some routinely, others by special request, enterable by terminal. A report can be with sexes separated or intermixed, and be ordered in various optional ways for any one department, including

- •by priority
- •by the local planning code
- •by date of registration in the waiting list
- •by critical date

and, relevant to use as a reception report,

- •by cited planned date of admission.

The choice is indicated by the department using the KPR or KPRO dialog, as discussed below.

Since a lengthy departmental waiting list brings difficulty in locating any particular patient, the above report is always accompanied by an alphabetical index of the patients, showing surname, PNR/RNR and line number for each - printed three to a row.

Besides the standard report above, three special reports of wait-listed patients are available

Special List #1, being as the standard list but excluding patients with priority code value I.

Special List #2, which the department is able to restrict to certain diagnoses or be sorted by diagnosis, is able to exclude priorities N and I.

Special List #3, covering patients with a critical date that falls within the coming 14 days.

Dialogs KPR & KPRO - requesting waiting-list reports

Use of KPR (for inpatient services) and KPRO (for outpatient services) plus identification of institution and department is the opening means for requesting reports of the departmental waiting lists.

Beyond the textual translation of the entered codes and the instruction to enter data or break, the form-display response comprises an array of six lines, for six different reports, and columns for specifying various characteristics, namely

- SPECIAL - indicating an explicit date when a report is required
- INTERVAL - being a number followed by D for days or M for months, expressing interval between recurrent issues
- DY - being the day (1st to 28th only) in the month for monthly etc., reports
- VM - a field provided initially to allow the above field to apply correspondingly to day of week, this field being D or M
- START - date for initial issue

STOP - date for final issue (to this specification)

Dialogs KPRP & KPRPO - requesting special waiting list #2

These two dialogs are similar to the preceding pair except that they deal with the more complicated options pertaining to Special Waiting List #2. The form-display with which the computer responds provides opportunity to request up to nine different lists each with its group of patients selected and/or ordered independently. For each line the central columns allow the specification of one value or a range of values of the department's planning code and/or the same for diagnosis code. The last column provides for a limit on the number of non-priority patients to be included; priorities FF and F are routinely included; the value in the last column limits those of N, I or P priority, selected in that order. Blank is taken as zero in this column.

Within each group the patients are ordered by the planning code or the diagnosis code value, as used.

If the same group number appears on two or more lines, the corresponding sets of patients are regarded as one group, to be included in one report. Otherwise each line used generates a separate report.

Dialogs VPLP & VPLPO - requesting of special issue of waiting list

These dialogs are similar to KPR and KPRO except that they are restricted to requesting a single issue of any report. They function identically except for having all columns after SPECIAL removed.

Statistical Reports

For each month and each department, a statistical report is issued, to show the overall status of the departmental list and its change over the month. Besides showing numbers of additions and deletions plus current total, if distinguishes the number of priority and high priority patients in each group. It also gives the number of high priority-patients that had to wait more than the intended six days, and the number of ordinary priority that had to wait more than the intended six weeks.

TRAFFIC LOAD

Table 6-1 provides an analysis of the telecommunications traffic within the Waiting List subsystem, together with an indication of consequential demands in the central computer. While almost twice as voluminous in transmission characters as the average dialog in the System, the load in the central computer per dialog is somewhat less than average. The Waiting List provides almost 10% of daily dialogs.

DIALOG	AVERAGE IMPACT PER DIALOG						DAILY TRAFFIC		
	TELECOMS		OTHER I/O		PROG	CPU			
	MSGS	CHARS	ACC	KWDS	CALLS	SECS	MIN	MEAN	MAX
VPL	5	2380	20	14	5	.44	221	348	517
VPLK	5	2021	15	11	4	.38	351	435	497
ETC									
OVERALL	5	1770	14	10	5	.33	1311	1530	1888

TABLE 6-1 REAL-TIME PROCESSING STATISTICS FOR WAITING LIST SUB-SYSTEM, BASED ON SURVEY 1 THRU 5 SEP 75.

(SEE TABLE 5-1 FOR EXPLANATIONS.)

CHAPTER 7

THE INPATIENT SUB-SYSTEM

While the focus of the inpatient sub-system is the record-keeping on a patient in hospital, the sub-system extends, by convenience, to include pre-admission activities relating to booked patients and, virtually of necessity, to post-discharge completion of the records.

Entry of a patient into this sub-system thus occurs either when a place is booked or when an unbooked patient is admitted to the hospital. (Like the P.R. with which it relates, and all the sub-systems other than waiting list, the inpatient sub-system is implemented independently for each hospital.) These two forms of entry clearly require different sequences of data entry, these being initiated by the PSV and ISV dialogs respectively.

PRE-ADMISSION

Dialog PSV - recording the booking of a patient for admission

Transmission of the message

PSV PNR/RNR

(inclusive or exclusive of the check digit) brings the form-response illustrated in Fig 7-1, with such entries completed as possible from the H.R.

```
¬¬¬¬¬¬¬¬¬¬¬¬¬¬¬¬¬¬¬¬¬¬¬¬¬¬¬¬¬¬¬¬¬¬¬¬¬¬¬¬¬¬¬¬¬¬¬¬¬¬¬¬¬¬¬¬¬¬¬¬¬¬¬¬¬¬¬¬¬¬¬¬¬¬
¬¬                                                                        ¬¬
¬¬ PSV 410101-0073                                                        ¬¬
¬¬ INPATIENT BED BOOKING                                                  ¬¬
¬¬ ENTER DATA OR BREAK                                                    ¬¬
¬¬ PNR  410101-0073                                                       ¬¬
¬¬ NAME  PETERSON, PETER HANS                                             ¬¬
¬¬ ADR  25 THE STRAND                                                     ¬¬
¬¬ ADMC       RINST ..... RDEPT ...  OI   .   BDAT 750611                 ¬¬
¬¬ INST ..... DEPT ...     CLN ...  PRTY ..  ACOD .                       ¬¬
¬¬ P1  ............... 2 ............... 3 ..................... ¬¬
¬¬ IDAT ...... ESTA ...   PCL   ..   SCOD .   ATN  .                      ¬¬
¬¬ ATS ....................................                               ¬¬
¬¬ PROC ...................... PRC ... OP ... DATE ......                 ¬¬
¬¬ PROC ...................... PRC ... OP ... DATE ......                 ¬¬
¬¬ PROC ...................... PRC ... OP ... DATE ......                 ¬¬
¬¬                                                                        ¬¬
¬¬                                                                        ¬¬
¬¬                                                                        ¬¬
¬¬¬¬¬¬¬¬¬¬¬¬¬¬¬¬¬¬¬¬¬¬¬¬¬¬¬¬¬¬¬¬¬¬¬¬¬¬¬¬¬¬¬¬¬¬¬¬¬¬¬¬¬¬¬¬¬¬¬¬¬¬¬¬¬¬¬¬¬¬¬¬¬¬
```

FIG 7-1 PSV - INITIAL COMPUTER RESPONSE

Following the repeated identification number, the T and N represent field names for telephone contact and nationality, the former accommodating the full number plus a code indicating whether the number is at work, home, or that of an intermediary. In the next line P stands for profession/occupation and CIV for civil status, the one allowing a textual answer, the other the standard 1-digit code. After the methodical address come the fields concerning the booking,

ADMC 1-digit (tentative) admission code, indicating whether patient is expected to be admitted from home, from another department of the same institution (transfers between departments are regarded as discharge-plus-admission) or from another institution

RINST 5-digit code of referring institution

RDEPT 3-digit code of referring department therein

OI a currently unused field

BDAT booking of date - entered automatically by computer

INST 5-digit code of institution in which booked

DEPT 3-digit code of department therein

PRTY 2-letter priority code

ACOD accommodation code - single, double or public room

P1 preliminary diagnosis - first

2 preliminary diagnosis - second

3 preliminary diagnosis - third

IDAT (admission) date i.e. planned one at this point

ESTA expected length of stay

PCL patient class

SCOD secrecy code; Y = yes implies special confidentiality

ATN admission tests - normal; Y = yes

ATS admission tests - special; textual entry

PROC, PRC, OP, DATE fields to allow specification of up to three procedures to be carried out - entries being procedure name and code, initials of desired operator and desired date. Not currently used.

Of these, BCOD, BDAT, INST, DEPT & IDAT must be entered, along with a usable address; the others are optional.

Transmission of the completed form-display leads as normal to data checking and consequential response from the computer, with depression of the REG key and transmission being the usual ending. However, to allow for late but immediate alteration, the data acceptance statement allows for alteration and rechecking of the data, by transmitting without any answer or use of a special key.

Dialogs PSVK - correction of admission booking

Transmission of PSVK plus a PNR/RNR brings display of the currently recorded booking data, just as it last appeared on a screen, and allows alteration of any fields other than INST, DEPT and IDAT. The procedure is essentially a repetition of PSV.

Dialog PSVU - obtaining information on booking

This dialog functions in the same manner as PSVK except that it is terminated automatically with the display of the current record, thereby prohibiting alteration.

ADMISSION

Dialogs ISV, ISVK & ISVU - the admitting record

These three dialogs parallel those of the PSV series but refer instead to the actual admission. An ISV is used to record the admission, an ISVK to alter that record, and an ISVU to obtain a sight of the record.

Transmission of ISV plus PNR/RNR initiates the basic dialog and brings a form-display to the screen. This is completed to the extent possible from the waiting list or, failing that, the H.R.

Following the patient's address and other data already discussed under dialog PSV, this display provides firstly room to identify the next-of-kin and append the appropriate address and telephone number. The subsequent fields that are extra to those of the PSV comprise

ACUT	whether the admission was acute; Y=yes
SIO	applicable State Insurance Office branch number
CTY	reference number of county of residence
MUN	reference number of municipality of residence (within county)
CLN	the 3-character code of the clinic/ward involved

At this juncture, the computer places the current date in IDAT, obliging the user to make an entry in this field only in exceptional cases.

No subsequent opportunity exists for amendment of this admission date. The ISVK dialog allows amendment of all others, except admitting institution, department and clinic/ward.

Where the P.R. contains more than one admission record for a patient, the ISVK and ISVU dialogs lead to the latest one if used as illustrated. However, inclusion of the appropriate admission date after PNR/RNR in the opening message leads to selection of the particular one.

TRANSFER AND PASS-OUT

Dialog PIK - recording of transfer within department

Reporting of the transfer of an inpatient from one ward to another is initiated by transmitting

PIK PNR/RNR

The response (assuming the System has the patient as currently admitted) has the date of transfer routinely filled by the computer but alterable by the user. Recording the transfer consists of entering the new ward identity in the indicated field, having the data accepted, then using the REG procedure.

Transfer of a patient between departments is regarded as discharge and admission - as already noted above.

Dialogs PP, PPK & PPU - permission to be on pass-out

Permission for an inpatient to be on pass-out for any significant period is reported using the PP dialog, amendable using the PPK dialog, and viewable using the PPU dialog. Opportunity exists to express the period as just between two dates, or more accurately by time. The procedures are comparable with those of the earlier trios, the date being included in the opening message of PPK and PPU where necessary.

Dialogs TTA & FTA - temporary transfer to a technical department

The transfer of a patient to an intensive care unit is regarded differently from a transfer between normal wards or normal clinical departments. An intensive care unit is regarded as a "technical" department, and the transfer thereto as essentially temporary, leaving the patient's normal accommodation still occupied. The TTA and FTA dialogs provide for such transfers to and from a technical department - and are usable also for radiology and other departments if it is desired to record formally the temporary change in responsibility. For both dialogs the computer response to the characteristic opening message gives the 'permanent' location but requires entry of the technical location, and adds a presumptive current date while requiring the time of the transfer to be entered.

DISCHARGE

Dialogs USV, USVK & USKU - discharge of an inpatient

Transmission of

USV PNR/RNR

in reference to a patient recorded as currently in the hospital brings the response that initiates recording of the patient's discharge.

The computer again presumes the current date as the effective one and makes an anticipatory entry - in this case as discharge date (DDAT). It also anticipates discharge to private home by placing 1 in the discharge code field (DCOD). Both these anticipatory entries must be altered as necessary, the latter having alternative values

2= discharge to another department within same institution
3= discharge to another institution
4= discharged dead, with autopsy
5= discharged dead, no autopsy

The remaining fields are optional, except that the discharge time (DTIME) must be entered for a death. Fields DINR and DDEPT allow recording of the discharge destination if another department of the County.

The dialogs USVK and USVU are used in the familiar way to alter and to view, respectively, a discharge record - the discharge date being added in the opening message to avoid any ambiguity.

Dialogs DIA & DIAK - the discharge diagnoses

The final diagnoses are entered, following a discharge, using the DIA dialog initially, and altered (or viewed) using DIAK, Fig 7-2 illustrating the response.

Either dialog must add the admission date to the PNR/RNR in the opening message, and must, of course, hit an appropriate discharge record. The tabular response to either provides columns labelled E-CD, DIAGNOSIS, CAUSE OF DEATH, OPDATE, OPNC, ANEC, the last three being tied together in any row, but the earlier ones being in independent columns.

The dialog DIA is illustrated, in Fig 7-3, after entry of values in

```
DIA  000101+0073  751024
DIAGNOSIS REPORTING - INPATNT DISCHARGE
ENTER DATA OR BREAK
PNR  000101+0073       NAME JACOBSON, PETER....................
INSTN 11002 DEPT  403  STN 601  DDAT 751024
 DIAGNOSIS CODES
 1 ...-..        2 ...-..          3 ...-..         4 ...-..
 5 ...-..        6 ...-..          7 ...-..         8 ...-..
 DNR  OPNC  OPDATE  ANEC         DNR  OPNC  OPDATE  ANEC
  .   ....  ......  ...-.         .   ....  ......  ...-.
  .   ....  ......  ...-.         .   ....  ......  ...-.
  .   ....  ......  ...-.         .   ....  ......  ...-.
  .   ....  ......  ...-.         .   ....  ......  ...-.
 E-CD   ....-. DNR .   TB .  TBBAC .   CAUSE OF D .          .
```

FIG 7-2 DIA - INITIAL RESPONSE.

```
DIA  000101+0073 751008
DIAGNOSIS REPORTING - INPATNT DISCHARGE  CLEARTEXT
ENTER F=FORWARD, R=RETURN TO DIA, B=BACK OR BREAK r
DIAGNOSIS 1          X         X
          E-CD       X         X
          OPERATION  X         X
          ANESTH     X         X
          OPERATION  X         X
          ANESTH     X         X
          OPERATION  X         X
DIAGNOSIS 2          X
          OPERATION  X         X
          ANESTH     X         X
DIAGNOSIS 3          X
```

FIG 7-3 DIA - CLEAR TEXT RESPONSE TO INPUT OF CODES.

these columns, completion of the acceptance phase and completion of the data registration phase - i.e. at the close of a successful dialog, when the entered codes have been automatically converted to text.

REPORTS OF FORTHCOMING ADMISSIONS

An important aspect of the inpatient sub-system is the facility it gives for advising various sections of the hospital, in advance, of expected admissions and their impending demands.

Each day Datacentral issues printed reports of the morrow's expected admissions in four styles

- for the receiving ward - showing the type of accommodation, the preliminary diagnoses, the tests to be done on admission, and any other procedures already noted; only the patients for the ward are listed, in PNR/RNR numeric order, and any pertinent critical medical data recorded on the H.R. is displayed alongside the other data.
- for the information desk - a similar report but lacking diagnoses and critical medical data, the patients being ordered lexicographically by name, across the total institution; the department and ward are shown alongside each patient's name.
- for the central laboratories - a report with the same contents as that to the ward; the patients are grouped into separate part-reports corresponding to each department, and ordered by PNR/RNR value therein.
- for the medical records department - a report similar in organization to that for the central laboratories but showing, beyond the number and name, only the ward for each patient.

In all these reports, which are necessarily more exposed to unwanted observation than a display on a terminal, the name of a patient is omitted if the special secrecy note had been made in the SLV/SLVK dialog process.

DIALOG	AVERAGE IMPACT PER DIALOG						DAILY TRAFFIC		
	TELECOMS		OTHER I/O		PROG	CPU			
	MSGS	CHARS	ACC	KWDS	CALLS	SECS	MIN	MEAN	MAX
POS	2	330	5	2	15	.08	706	902	1186
ISV	5	1762	31	15	15	.47	485	682	692
USV	5	1045	18	8	10	.26	445	538	651
PIK	5	820	20	8	11	.23	104	132	195
DIA	5	1573	15	13	6	.28	264	384	605
ETC									
OVERALL	4	1081	17	9	9	.26	2515	2922	3194

TABLE 7-1 REAL-TIME PROCESSING STATISTICS FOR INPATIENT SUB-SYSTEM, BASED ON SURVEY 1 THRU 5 SEP 75.

(SEE TABLE 5-1 FOR EXPLANATIONS.)

TRAFFIC LOAD

Table 7-1 provides an analysis of the telecommunications traffic within the inpatient sub-system, together with an indication of consequential demands in the central computer. As Table 5-1 shows, the daily traffic of this sub-system accounts for about 18% of System dialogs. However, while this component is a little higher per dialog than average in characters transferred to and from terminals, it is lower than average in most central computer pressures. Table 7-1 shows successively lower numbers of POS, ISV, USV and DIA dialog groupings; this is due to declining need for amendments from pre-admission to post-discharge.

CHAPTER 8

THE BOOKING SUB-SYSTEM

The booking sub-system relates to the booking of outpatient appointments - to family practice units, specialty clinics and service departments. With its simultaneous aims of improved response to patient needs and desires, and improved utilization of facilities, the application is seen as of major potential in the beneficial adaptation of computers to health care.

The sub-system was designed for use by receptionists and booking clerks, often if not usually with the patient in close attendance. However, as adverted to earlier, it was not designed ab initio within the framework of the overall County system, but was adapted from a pioneering development of the Karolinska hospital.

The P.R. is again the key section of the data base for the application, this time in the form of the DBP and VL files plus the HP file, the DBP record being the explicit booking record. The H.R. is as usual a potential source of what otherwise would be key-entered data, and in return can acquire telephone numbers gained in the booking process, but is otherwise unconcerned with this sub-system.

Beyond the patient-oriented files, the booking sub-system demands files of the resources that can be booked, and of the services they provide. This requires both the recording of data on operating hours and the continuous maintenance by the computer of appointment commitments. The sub-system has been built to allow considerable variety in the patterns of operation, including even special priority sessions and double booking. Even the recording of the operational data is a real-time process, allowing immediate adjustment of files in response to operational changes.

The reports emanating from the sub-system batch programs include routine advanced listings of appointments.

MAKING BOOKINGS

The sub-system was designed on the principle that the receptionist or booking clerk enters the needs and the computer responds with three alternative times for each, with the option to the user of seeking further alternatives if desired.

Dialog BOKA - booking appointments

The basic dialog of the sub-system is BOKA, which is initiated by the message

BOKA PNR/RNR

the response to which is illustrated in Fig 8-1 (for a case where the computer had record of the patient's name).

After the fields for coded entry of hospital, department and station from which the case is being referred, plus a short field for entry of free

```
-------------------------------------------------------------------------
--                                                                     --
-- BOKA  170312+1234  BOOKING APPOINTMENTS                             --
--                                                                     --
--  PNR/RNR 170312+1234  NAME ANDERSON, ERIK CARL ROLF                 --
--  REGISTERING INSTITN  11002       DEPT  ...     STN  ...            --
--  REFERRED FROM .............                                        --
-- EXAMINATION/RESOURCE                                                --
--     E1/R1 .... ....  E2/R2 .... ....  E3/R3 .... ....  INT ..      --
--     E1/R1 .... ....  E2/R2 .... ....  E3/R3 .... ....  INT ..      --
--     E1/R1 .... ....  E2/R2 .... ....  E3/R3 .... ....              --
--                                                                     --
-- EXAMINATION DATE     EARLIEST ......  LATEST  ......                --
-- EXCLUDED INTERVAL     ...... - ...... PCLASS  .                     --
--                                                                     --
--                                                                     --
--                                                                     --
--                                                                     --
--                                                                     --
-------------------------------------------------------------------------
```

FIG 8-1 BOKA - INITIAL DISPLAY.

text concerning the reference, the form display proceeds to specification of the needed appointments.

The three repetitious lines provide space for the entry of up to nine needed appointments, grouped as three groups of three. Each row represents a group of up to three appointments to be made for a single day, the symbolic pairs E1/R1, E2/R2, and E3/R3 each calling for a 4-digit code for service and, optionally, a 3-digit code for a particular facility. The former may be a general visit, an x-ray or so on, either investigational or therapeutic; as discussed earlier, it has been accorded the generic name 'examination' in this text, hence the 'E' shown in this display. The abbreviation EXAM is used for the corresponding code in Appendix B, and in displays that allow the space. The shorter code refers to 'RESOURCE', which is also covered in Appendix B; the code values identify machines in some departments, rooms in others, people in yet others. Normally this field is left blank, allowing the choice to be made automatically according to the circumstances.

The provision of the second and third lines of this array allows either the requesting of more than three examinations or a requesting of explicit spacing of different (groups of) examinations on different days. Such spacing is achieved by using the field INT at the end of each of the first two lines in the array; those apply respectively to the spacing from first to second and from second to third groups. The appropriate code values and their meanings in a particular situation are:-

blank	the two groups are to be on separate days, but with no particular spacing otherwise, and in either order
1 thru 99	the two groups are to be on dates that differ at least by the value shown, and in the order shown
0	the 'overflow' situation; the two groups can be on the same day.

Differential use of the two available INT fields thus allows up to six examinations to be sought for one day and three for another, as well as up to nine on a single day or up to three on each of three distinct days. And, where separate dates are demanded for separate groups, it can be either merely to avoid undue pressure on any one day or to achieve an explicit spacing and sequence for medical reasons.

The penultimate line in the display provides opportunity to delimit the calendar interval within which the examinations should be fitted, default implying "as soon as possible". The final line allows, on the contrary, the exclusion of a calendar interval (e.g. because of the patient expecting to be on vacation, or in hospital) and, finally, scope for specifying a priority for the patient. Only one level of abnormal priority is identified, denoted by 'Y', and carries the privilege in certain departments of being allowed a booking in special reserved booking periods.

```
BOKA  170312+1234  BOOKING APPOINTMENTS

 PNR/RNR 170312+1234  NAME ANDERSON, ERIK CARL ROLF
 REGISTERING INSTITN  11002        DEPT ...       STN ...
 REFERRED FROM   DR JOHNS....
EXAMINATION/RESOURCE
    E1/L1 0622 7330  E2/R2 0637 7331  E3/R3 .... ....  INT ..
    E1/L1 0450 ....  E2/R2 .... ....  E3/R3 .... ....  INT ..
    E1/L1 1011 ....  E2/R2 .... ....  E3/R3 .... ....

EXAMINATION DATE     EARLIEST  ...... LATEST  ......
EXCLUDED INTERVAL      ...... - ...... PCLASS  .
```

FIG 8-2 BOKA - SUBMISSION OF NEEDS.

The computer checks the acceptability of the data entered as specification of the needs before proceeding to any selection of possibilities for the appointments.

Given an error-free message, e.g. as in Fig 8-2, the computer seeks three alternative (sets of) times for presentation to the booking clerk, within the criteria and constraints specified. Examinations grouped on one line in the requesting message remained grouped on a line in all offering messages, with three alternative groups of appointments being offered, but with each group being an unalterable set of appointments within a single day. Each display shows the date at the left, then the one, two or three appointments in the form of time plus abbreviated name (interpreted from the submitted codes) and finally the total elapsed time that the appointment(s) should span.

Fig 8-3 illustrates a possible response to the message of Fig 8-2, and shows how the three groups of preferred appointments are assembled as three blocks, each with the same array as that of the requesting message. (Rather, for instance, than in chronological order of offerings or with alternatives for any group adjacent.)

```
----------------------------------------------------------------------
--                                                                  --
-- BOKA  170312+1234  ANDERSON, ERIK CARL ROLF                      --
-- BOOKING ALTERNATIVES                                             --
-- ANSWER OR BREAK                          r 1 3 2             r --
--    11 APR 0925 THOR'C SPI  1010  HAND              T 1;10        --
--    10 APR 0825 GALLBLADDE                          T 0;45        --
--    17 APR 1105 RETURN VIS                          T 0;55        --
--                                                                  --
--    12 APR 0855 THOR'C SPI  0955  HAND              T 1;25        --
--    11 APR 0825 GALLBLADDE                          T 0;45        --
--    18 APR 1000 RETURN VIS                          T 0;55        --
--                                                                  --
--    17 APR 0855 THOR'C SPI  0955  HAND              T 1;25        --
--    13 APR 0840 GALLBLADDE                          T 0;45        --
--    20 APR 1000 RETURN VIS                          T 0;55        --
-- PLEASE CHECK THAT THE ANSWER MEETS THE SEQUENCE                  --
-- CONSTRAINTS SPECIFIED IN THE REQUEST                             --
--                                                                  --
----------------------------------------------------------------------
```

FIG 8-3 BOKA INITIAL OFFERING OF ALTERNATIVE APPOINTMENTS.

(ACTUALLY SHOWN AFTER INSERTION OF SELECTIONS BY USER.)

The request contained two examinations in the first group, and these can be seen paired each time and as producing a varying elapsed time as their respective clock times change relatively. The request also required that the third examination group be at least five days after the second, but left the first arbitrary. In the blocks offered it happens that the first-listed group follows the second in each case.

The user chooses by entering digits in the normal answer zone. Fig 8-3 shows such digits, namely 1 3 2, already in place, i.e. it illustrates the computer offering after entry of the user's choice, these character positions being blank initially. The three digits represent the ordinal choice of the successive groups; the '3' represents the choice of the third alternative offered for the second-listed group (i.e. the "GALLBLADDE") for example.

Clearly, from this example, it can be seen that the user does not have to choose in toto one computer-proffered block. Since the computer does not repeat any one alternative, it follows that, beyond the first block being the earliest possible assemblage, no special association applies to the members of a block beyond them being compatible with the specified relationships and constraints. And it is, of course, because selections from two or more blocks do not necessarily even meet such conditions that the exhortation appears at the foot of the screen.

Transmission of the message brings a similar display in response, but with the chosen lines denoted by leading asterisks and row 3 containing the statement

DATA ACCEPTED, RESPOND REG, REGCPR, REGCEN OR BREAK

the details of which are explained below.

If no suitable combination of appointments can be obtained from the initial array of offerings, additional alternatives can be elicited by inserting letters in place of digits in the user-answer zone. Working on the basis that additional alternatives imply later alternatives, the user is given the option, for each examination group, of entering A, B or C to signify respectively that the new set of alternatives is to start from the date of the first, second or third of the currently displayed set for that group. Thus, for instance, a response B C C to the offerings of Fig 8-3 would imply new alternatives for the thoracic and hand x-rays starting 12APR, for the gall-bladder x-ray starting 13APR and for the return visit starting 20APR.

```
--                                                                    --
-- BOKA  170312+1234  ANDERSON, ERIK CARL ROLF                        --
-- BOOKING ALTERNATIVES                                               --
-- ANSWER OR BREAK                              r                   r --
-- NEW ALTERNATIVES - GROUP 1                                         --
--   12 APR 0900 THOR'C SPI  0955  HAND                T 1;20         --
--   17 APR 0855 THOR'C SPI  0955  HAND                T 1;25         --
--   17 APR 0925 THOR'C SPI  1010  HAND                T 1;10         --
-- NEW ALTERNATIVES - GROUP 2                                         --
--   13 APR 0845 GALLBLADDE                            T 0;45         --
--   14 APR 0825 GALLBLADDE                            T 0;45         --
--   14 APR 0835 GALLBLADDE                            T 0;45         --
-- NEW ALTERNATIVES - GROUP 3                                         --
--   20 APR 1005 RETURN VIS                            T 0;55         --
--   20 APR 1025 RETURN VIS                            T 0;55         --
--   20 APR 1045 RETURN VIS                            T 0;55         --
--                                                                    --
--                                                                    --
```

FIG 8-4 BOKA - ADDITIONAL APPOINTMENT ALTERNATIVES.

Fig 8-4 shows the response of the computer to such an answer. It should be noted that, at this stage, the computer desists from assembling the alternatives in blocks, but merely lists the three lines of alternatives adjacently for each group. This is due to the fact that a different density of availabilities for the different examinations would, if potential appointments were maintained in blocks consistent with the criteria, result in many potential times remaining obscured.

Again the digits 1, 2 and 3 are used to denote the choosing of the first, second or third alternative offered for any one group, and entered in sequence in the answer zone. If any set is still inadequate, the relevant digit position can have an 'F' entered in it to denote "further alternatives required". The computer then proceeds to offer a further set for each so-denoted group while simultaneously displaying the choices that have been made. Assuming 1 2 F as the user response to Fig 8-4, the next display could be as in Fig 8-5. The procedure is repeated as necessary, until a full block of choices has been made, at which point the DATA ACCEPTED... statement is obtained together with the listing, under CHOSEN ALTERNATIVES, of all the choices.

The combining of letters and digits, illustrated in the last cited user response, can be adopted from the outset as regards the A, B and C. Thus, instead of 1 3 2 or B C C such responses as 1 2 C can be given to signify partial satisfaction with the initial offerings.

```
--------------------------------------------------------------------------
--                                                                       --
-- BOKA  170312+1234  ANDERSON, ERIK CARL DANIEL                         --
-- BOOKING ALTERNATIVES                                                  --
-- ANSWER OR BREAK                                      r              r --
-- CHOSEN ALTERNATIVES                                                   --
--   12 APR 0900  THOR'C SPI 0955  HAND X                    T 1;20      --
--   14 APR 0825 GALLBLADDE                                  T 0;45      --
--                                                                       --
-- NEW ALTERNATIVES - GROUP 3                                            --
--   20 APR 1050  RETURN VIS                                 T 0;55      --
--   20 APR 1105  RETURN VIS                                 T 0;55      --
--   20 APR 1110  RETURN VIS                                 T 0;55      --
--                                                                       --
--                                                                       --
--                                                                       --
--                                                                       --
--                                                                       --
--                                                                       --
--------------------------------------------------------------------------
```

FIG 8-5 BOKA - CHOSEN AND NEW ALTERNATIVES.

If, on the other hand, a plethora of alternatives in a relatively undesirable time period seems to be available, or other reason exists, the user can always BREAK and re-start with adjusted constraints.

The alternatives REG, REGCPT & REGCEN offered in the DATA ACCEPTED... message all denote acceptance of the block of bookings by the user. The differences relate to written notification for the patient, REGCPT initiating the displaying of a message suitable for printing on the associated character printer, and REGCEN calling for the printing and despatch of a similar message by Datacentral; REG alone abjures such notification message. Fig 8-6 illustrates the written advice, while further

```
HUDDINGE HOSPITAL NOTIFICATION OF BOOKINGS MADE ON 4/APR/76
***    APPOINTMENTS MADE FOR YOU AT HUDDINGE HOSPITAL    ***
NAME  ANDERSON, ERIK CARL ROLF
ADR   33 CHESTNUT AV.              31760  TABY
TEL   NONE
THIS NOTICE APPLIES TO THE TIMES AND LOCATIONS LISTED BELOW
TOGETHER WITH INSTRUCTIONS CONCERNING THE VISIT. IF YOU ARE
UNABLE TO ATTEND, PLEASE ADVISE HOSPITAL  TEL 08/746 1000
TIME      DATE

0900    12 APR 1976  THOR'C SPI    SEE INSTRUCTION #3, #5
                                   X-RAY DEPT.
0955    12 APR 1976  HAND
                                   X-RAY DEPT
0825    14 APR 1976  GALLBLADDE    SEE INSTRUCTION #3
                                   X-RAY DEPT
1105    20 APR 1976  RETURN VIS
                                   GASTROENT DEPT.
```

FIG 8-6 THE BOOKING ADVICE TO THE PATIENT.

discussion of appointment advices is include below under BOKBA.

At this point the computer proceeds to display such other data as

```
--------------------------------------------------------------------------
--                                                                      --
-- BOKA  180312+1233                                                    --
-- BOOKING ALTERNATIVES                                                 --
-- ENTER DATA OR BREAK                          r                    r --
-- PNR/RNR  180312+1233  NAME  ANDERSON, ERIK CARL ROLF........        --
-- TEL       NONE....... NAT  ..   SEX M      OCCP JOINER              --
-- ADR 33 CHESTNUT AV...........    PONR 31740 PA TABY                 --
--                                                                      --
--                                                                      --
--                                                                      --
--                                                                      --
--                                                                      --
--                                                                      --
--                                                                      --
--                                                                      --
--                                                                      --
--                                                                      --
--                                                                      --
--------------------------------------------------------------------------
```

FIG 8-7 BOKA - PERSONAL REGISTRATION DETAILS.

address and telephone number, to the extent that it has such data for the cited patient, and seeks its correction/completion. Fig 8-7 illustrates this display of basic registration data - the entry NONE alongside TEL indicating no telephone available or known. After any alteration and then checking, this information is registered in the P.R. If the patient is already in the P.R. for the relevant institution all the registration data should be available. If the patient is not in the P.R., but is in H.R. through being a resident of the County, all but perhaps telephone should be available, but there may be a need to update some fields (although no such updating of H.R. can be achieved except through advice from the central authorities). If the patient is in neither the H.R. nor the P.R., an automatic coupling is made to the OPVP dialog (q.v. Chapter 9).

The computer makes a tentative reservation of every appointment alternative prior to it being offered to the user via the display - i.e. makes three reservations for each examination requested. The selection of one alternative results in its firm reservation; the rejected two have their tentative reservations withdrawn, as do any alternatives rejected by the seeking of others. Hence there is no chance of a proffered alternative becoming unavailable during the time the particular user is considering it, but, correspondingly, there is advantage in recording each selection as quickly as possible.

MANUALLY EFFECTED BOOKING

Where a breakdown of the System or the desire to pursue a non-standard practice (e.g. double-booking or booking outside scheduled hours) precludes use of the BOKA dialog, licence exists to make bookings outside of the computer processes. However, if appropriate records are to be maintained in adequate condition and, after major breakdown, chaos is to be avoided in future bookings, the externally effected bookings must be advised to the computer as soon as possible. This is effected using the BOKM dialog.

```
-------------------------------------------------------------------------
--                                                                     --
-- BOKM  183012+1233                                                   --
-- REGISTRATION OF MANUALLY EFFECTED BOOKING                           --
-- ENTER NEW DATA, REG OR BREAK                    r                 r --
--  PNR/RNR  180312+1233  NAME  ANDERSON, ERIK CARL ROLF               --
--  REGISTERING INSTITN  11002 DEPT ...  CLN ...                       --
--  REFERRED FROM   DR.JOHNS....    BOOKING DATE  760228               --
--                                                                     --
--  E-1 0622 RESOURCE 7330 DATE 760412 ARRIVE 0900 START               --
--  E-2 0455 RESOURCE 7310 DATE 760414 ARRIVE 0840 START               --
--  E-3 .... RESOURCE .... DATE ...... ARRIVE .... START               --
--                                                                     --
--                                                                     --
--                                                                     --
--                                                                     --
--                                                                     --
--                                                                     --
--                                                                     --
-------------------------------------------------------------------------
```

FIG 8-8 BOKM - ENTRY DATA.

Dialog BOKM - recording a manually effected booking

Transmission of
BOKM PNR/RNR
brings a form-display response for entry of the data relating to the one or more bookings that have been made for the cited patient. Fig 8-8 illustrates this after entry of various data. The various fields are either self-explanatory or similar to those of BOKA. The booking date is presumptively entered by the computer, but is alterable. The last field on each repeated line is for automatic entry of the effective start time, based on the entered arrival time and the examination involved; it is not currently used.

As with BOKA, following registration of the booking data the BOKM dialog continues with messages concerning the personal data of the patient.

The non-standard practices of double booking and booking outside scheduled hours clearly present hazards to the overall operations, and technical problems for the computer records. Since no such practice can reasonably be resorted to without the concurrence of the serving department, the System only accepts such anomalies when the serving department is the department making the booking.

Double-booking and even outside-hours booking can be done inadvertently during periods of breakdown. Whether deliberate or inadvertent, such anomalies bring an exception response following the data-checking phase. Below the entered data, each such anomaly is identified as to the appointment (by 'E-1', 'E-2', etc.,) then the transgression. Anwering with 'BOK' in the answer zone, instead of the routine registration procedure, will bypass those controls if the department code is satisfactory.

ANCILLARY BOOKING DIALOGS

Having entered a booking and arranged for the patient to be advised, subsequent need for observing a patient's bookings and for a new advice to the patient may arise; dialogs BOKU and BOKBA provide for these needs. The former of these also provides the means for cancelling any recorded booking.

The dialog BOKK allows addition, viewing, and alteration of a free-text commentary field that can be attached to any booking.

Dialog BOKU - observing and cancelling booking records

The input message
BOKU PNR/RNR
prompts display of a patient's bookings, in the manner illustrated in Fig 8-9. This is a chronological listing of all booking records currently in the P.R. for the cited patient, even though older records may relate to dates past, at least to the extent of screen-capacity. (Any overflow is indicated by 'CONTD' at the foot of the screen, and can be reached by the usual procedure.)

```
BOKU  180312+1233   ANDERSON, ERIK CARL ROLF
BOOKED EXAMINATIONS
ENTER NEW DATA OR BREAK
EXAMINATION     PLACE   EXAM DATE     ARR  REFERRED   BOOKED CAN
THOR'C SPINE    SKEL    11 APR 1976   0925 DR.JOHNS   760404  .
HAND            SKEL1   11 APR 1976   1010 DR.JOHNS   760404  .
THOR'C SPINE    SKEL    12                                    .
HAND            SKEL1   12                                    .
GALLBLADDER     ALTRA   13                                    .
RETURN VISIT    MED 5   18                                    .
```

FIG 8-9 BOKU - INITIAL COMPUTER RESPONSE.

The right-hand column, headed 'CAN', provides for cancellations, the user signifying the pertinent bookings by entering 'C' = Cancel in the rows concerned. Any cancellations must pass through the checking phase and be registered; otherwise, if observation alone is required, the user merely breaks the dialog.

Dialog BOKBC - obtaining an appointment's advice

The BOKBC dialog provides the equivalent of a late 'REGCPT' response to a BOKA registration step, bringing forth essentially the same display except that, whereas the BOKA display covered only bookings being made by that dialog, the BOKBA message brings forth all bookings currently recorded. There is thus an increased likelihood of overflowing the screen; if this happens, the first screenful must be printed to completion then the next one called, by the usual procedure. As explained in Chapter 5, there is no trace of this discontinuity in the printed output.

```
BOKK    000101+0073  PETERSON, PETER
BOOKED EXAMINATION
ALTER/ADD COMMENTS, B=BACK, F=FORWARD, BREAK r                    r
   EXAM/TRTMNT      RES      APPT DATE  ARR  REFERED FR  B-DATE
   NEW VISIT        LEE    10 MAR 1976 0930 DR.BERG      760305
    1013  SEE LETTER OF 9 MAR...      ......................
   LUNGXRA          XRD 2 10 MAR 1976       DR.BERG      760305
    7114  PATNT WHEELCHAIR-BOUND      ......................
   CONTROLL         LEE    25 MAR 1976      MED CLIN     760310
    1020  ......................      ......................
```

FIG 8-10 BOKK - INITIAL RESPONSE.

Dialog BOKK - additional comments in the booking record

The one dialog BOKK allows the entry, perusal, alteration and removal of free text comment with each booking record. The initiating message cites only PNR/RNR after the dialog code, so obtains all bookings within the capacity of the screen. Fig 8-10 provides an example of this response, and shows how two 22-position fields are associated with each booking. Any comments already recorded are displayed, with marking dots completing the fields. Any of these character positions can be altered and the revised display transmitted back without entry in the answer zone, acceptance and registration of which will cause over-writing of extant comments.

INFORMATION ON CAPACITIES AND COMMITMENTS

The KAP series - capacity for appointments.

While the essential purpose of the booking application relates to the obtaining of appointments for patients, the overall management of the service facilities requires knowledge of forthcoming availabilities. To meet such needs various dialogs are available that provide large or small pictures of free capacity. These comprise

- KAP — hour-by-hour free capacity of a facility over a 10-day period
- KAPD — booking-interval free capacity of a facility over a single day

KAPM, KAPDM same as KAP and KAPD respectively, except that they take cognigance of the specified operating hours

Initiation of any of the four is essentially the same, being transmittal of the message

dialog R̲E̲S̲O̲U̲R̲C̲E̲ date

where the first represents dialog code, the second the code for the facility and the date is the (opening) date of the period to be displayed.

The response for KAP is illustrated in Fig 8-11, the facility being shown by abbreviated name as well as code in row 2. The successive columns of the array show the free capacity for the successive hours of the day e.g. between 07:00 and 08:00 hrs, while the lines are given an explicit sequence number as well as showing the dates.

The line numbers are referred to in the instructions of row 3, entry of any one in the answer zone leading to the detailed display, for the pertinent date, available otherwise through KAPD.

```
KAP 1310 760426
FREE CAPACITY FOR 7310 ALTRA
ENTER LINE-NR FOR DETAILS OR BREAK
                  07 08 09 10 11 12 13 14 15 16 17 18 19
  1  26 APR       60 60          30 60 60
  2  27 APR       60 45 45 30    30 60
  3  28 APR       60 50          30
  4  01 MAY       60 60 60 60    60
  5  02 MAY       60 30    30    30
  6  03 MAY       60 60          60
  7  04 MAY       60 45 15 30    60
  8  05 MAY       60 50 30 30    60
  9  08 MAY       60 50 30       60
 10  09 MAY       60 60    60    60
```

F̲I̲G̲ 8-11 KAP - DISPLAY OF GROSS FREE CAPACITY OVER DAYS.

The scheme for R̲E̲S̲O̲U̲R̲C̲E̲ is oriented to identifying single-patient facilities. Hence 60 minutes free in an hour means totally free, while lesser figures indicate the intrusion of one or more appointments. The figure '30' in a CAP display thus indicates a complementary booking of 30 minutes; however, it gives no indication of which particular parts of the hours are free. The KAPD display, illustrated in Fig 8-12, provides this information by citing each time that the facility becomes free (within the day concerned) and the duration it remains free. Thus, for instance, it shows whether 45 minutes available in one hour is continuous with some availability in an adjacent hour.

Unlike previously discussed dialogs in the booking application, this display with KAPD offers no choices to the user and has no potential for consequential computer action. With its issuance, therefore, the computer automatically closes the dialog - which fact it states in the last line.

Both KAP and KAPD report on the basis of a facility being operated continuously from 07:00 hrs to 19:00 hrs. every weekday. However, not only do many facilities operate a shorter day than this, but many specialty clinics operate for only a few hours per week. The actual specified operating hours are, of course, recorded in the System for booking purposes. The dialogs KAPM and KAPDM take cognizance of this, and recognize only availabilities within the specified times. Otherwise they function just like KAP and KAPD respectively.

```
-----------------------------------------------------------------------
--                                                                   --
-- KAPD 7310 760429                                                  --
-- FREE CAPACITY FOR 7310 ALTRA  27 APR 1976                         --
-- TIME  CAP                                  r               r      --
-- 0700   90                                                         --
-- 0845   15                                                         --
-- 0915   45                                                         --
-- 1030   30                                                         --
-- 1130  450                                                         --
--                                                                   --
--                                                                   --
-- FREE CAPACITY DISPLAYED. DIALOG CLOSED                            --
--                                                                   --
--                                                                   --
--                                                                   --
--                                                                   --
--                                                                   --
--                                                                   --
-----------------------------------------------------------------------
```

FIG 8-12 KAPD - DISPLAY OF GROSS FREE CAPACITY WITHIN A DAY.

SCHEDULES OF APPOINTMENTS

The accumulated diary of appointments for each day is printed overnight, a day in advance, in both a locally consolidated departmental/clinic form for each reception point and in a fully dissected form for the individual RESOURCE code values. The patients are listed in chronological order for attendance, with the following information for each

- planned arrival time
- examination, by short name
- RESOURCE
- PNR/RNR
- surname, limited amount of forename(s)
- telephone or inpatient location
- textual reference note
- intended departure time
- next appointment time and service, if any that day.

Separate listings of impending appointments are prepared for medical records staff, with the patients separated by department concerned, then listed in the order used for record storage, i.e. day then month then year of birth. The information shown for each patient is

PNR/RNR
surname, etc.
planned arrival time
examination, by short name
RESOURCE
textual reference note
note as to which of KRM, RTG and SV records are already in H.R.

Dialog BARK - daily list of late bookings

Since the above listings are produced a full day in advance of the operational day concerned, some late changes are to be expected for many service units. The BARK dialog produces a display of bookings made during the current day for the following (business) day. Transmission of the mere dialog code prompts listing over the whole of the user's institution, but the addition of a DEPT value restricts the list to the nominated department. The list is in numerical order of PNR/RNR, and its line layout is close to that of the latter of the above-described schedules.

Dialog AKTB - listing of bookings for a facility

The entry message
AKTB RESOURCE date
for a given value of RESOURCE code and date initiates a listing of all current bookings for the indicated resource and date. Fig 8-13 illustrates the response, which provides a chronological listing of all bookings, with each identified as to time, examination required, and patient concerned. (While earlier examples gave a suggestion of RESOURCE being subservient to EXAM, it must be recognized that a given resource can be used for more than one type of examination. Use of a general examining room for a succession of specialty clinics is an obvious example, the operation by one doctor of separate different specialty clinics another.)

Row 2 provides the short name of the designated location, while the succeeding rows offer a considerable range of responses for the user's choosing.

Since the screen can display a maximum of 10 appointments, the facility to turn on is available - namely entry of 'F' for 'forward' in the answer zone and transmission. (The NEXT-PAGE function key can be used equivalently. The availability of F and B here merely reflect early development.) The existence of more appointments on the day is shown by 'CONTD' in the last row. To reverse this procedure, 'B' for 'backward' is also available to the user. Processing of 'F' and 'B' is not in fact constrained by the date, and allows the user to look forward or back progressively through adjacent days.

A more selective revision of the listing can be obtained by answering with 'AM' or 'PM', which indicate an interest restricted to morning or to afternoon. Subsequent use of F or B is interpreted within this constraint.

Occurrence of a patient in a booking list can give rise to questions regarding the same patient's other appointments, e.g. whether some other

```
AKTB 1010 760916
BOOKED PATIENTS FOR X-SKEL   ABOVE DATE
ENTER DATA, BREAK OR LINK TO BOKU=LINE NR
PAGING FORWARD=F, BACK=B, MORNING=AM, AFTERNOON=PM.
NR TIME  EXAM  PNR/RNR     NAME                          N=NO SHOW
 1 0830  1020 030505-1237 JAROLIM, ANTON                        .
 2 1000  1019 631212-4014 HYTTANDER, DANIEL                     .
 3 1310  1020 240812-1222 BENGTSEN, BIRGITTA                    .
```

FIG 8-13 AKTB - INITIAL RESPONSE.

examination has been ordered or will have been completed, or whether other appointments on the same day allow or may cause variation of the appointment at the clinic concerned. Provision has, therefore, been made for automatically stepping from this dialog to BOKU, through entry in the answer zone of the line number of the patient appointment concerned. When the BOKU dialog is broken, the AKTB dialog is resumed at the point preceding departure.

The AKTB dialog is also the means for recording the non-attendance of a patient for an appointment, an 'N' in the indicated final column being the means, followed by the normal transaction registration procedure. Similar use of 'A' allows a reported no-show to be withdrawn.

MAINTAINING THE BASIC RESOURCE RECORDS

It is clear from the foregoing discussion of the booking procedures that elaborate information is required in the System regarding facilities, the services they provide, their operating schedules, and so on. The provision of this information to the computer can be effected by batch input or via terminal, the former means having been valuable at implementation time for any major new area, but the terminal means being the natural one for continuing maintenance, and even for significant expansion in an environment so attuned to real-time computing. In the following discussion attention will be, therefore, restricted to the real-time means for all aspects of creating and maintaining these basic records of the booking sub-system.

Four distinct facets can be recognised to these records

- the catalog of EXAM codes and their meanings
- the catalog of RESOURCE codes and their meanings
- the interrelationships of EXAM and RESOURCE codes, i.e. which EXAM codes are accommodated by each RESOURCE code value
- the operating timetable for each pairing of EXAM and RESOURCE

Four separate dialogs are provided to cover these four facets, these being respectively BUND, BRES, BRUK and BOM. These are used both for building the records for a new area of implementation, and for fragmentary maintenance thereafter.

Dialog BUND - building the EXAM catalog

Transmission of
BUND DEPT
brings a listing of all EXAM code values currently cataloged for the cited DEPT, together with associated data. Opportunity then exists to alter an existing one or add another, but the opportunity is limited to just one such action per dialog. To this purpose the display includes one blank line and one column, labelled 'D/A', wherein any existing code can be marked 'D' = Delete or 'A' = Alter.

The fields following the code value comprise a 16-character name field for the examination, a 21-character note field, the date of introduction of the examination into the sub-system, and a column allowing the denoting of the association of one of the pre-set standard comments. The name entered is the one used in the computer responses during the foregoing dialogs; the associated note appears alongside the name in the notification to the patient, together with the standard comment, if any, denoted.

Besides the restriction to one line so far as user entry is concerned, the deletion of an examination that is coupled to any resource is prohibited, because of the obvious difficulties this would cause. Any attempt to delete such an examination results in an advisory response that shows the resources coupled to the examination; and opportunity to delete all these by the normal registration process. Then the intended deletion of the examination can be completed.

If a new examination is entered, it is accorded its code value by the computer, being the lowest free value of the block assigned to the department concerned. In any future print-out or display, it appears in its numerical place.

The set of examinations performed by one department can easily exceed one screenful. Irrespective of this, one blank line for a new entry is always displayed. The existence of additional lines to the present screen display is advertised by the usual 'CONTD' at the foot, and they are accessed by the usual means.

Dialog BRES - building the RESOURCE catalog

This dialog functions in much the same way as BUND. The name accommodated for each resource is contracted to a mere five characters, while the comment field is used for the location (organizational or physical, as appropriate) to which the patient needs to be directed. Subsequent to these textual fields, three similar columns are provided for identifying the attendance schedules in which patients of the resource should be listed. The last column records the number of weeks in advance that the resource is bookable.

One other column is additional to the display in BUND, namely the line number. This is usable for stepping into a display of the couplings of the particular resource to the examinations. As with BUND, a coupled code cannot be deleted, but this branching into a display of couplings allows their cancellation and then deletion of the resource concerned.

In other respects BRES is just as BUND, allowing one insertion, deletion or altered line per dialog.

Dialog BRUK - coupling EXAM and RESOURCE catalogs

The coupling of EXAM and RESOURCE code values - i.e. the recording of which resources perform which examination services - is established, and can be observed, or altered, via the BRUK dialog. The initial message must cite DEPT then RESOURCE, and brings a response as illustrated in Fig 8-14.

```
BRUK  246 2410 COUPLING REPORT FOR RESOURCE 2410 LEE    DEPT 246
DELETE=D, ALTER=A
          ENTER DATA OR BREAK
 FOLLOWING EXAMINATIONS ARE COUPLED TO THE RESOURCE
        EXAM   PREP'N  EXAMINA-  POST             EXAM
   P/A  CODE    TIME  TION TIME EX TIME EFFDAT  NAME
    .   2402    10.      20.       5.   760317  NEW VISIT......
    .   2420    10.      20.       5.   760224  RETURN VISIT...
    .   ....    ....     ....     ....  ......  ...............
```

FIG 8-14 BRUK - INITIAL RESPONSE.

Again the singular option exists of deleting one line, altering one line, or inserting one new line, the style of operation being as in BUND and BRES. The only amenable fields are the three time fields - citing the number of minutes to be allowed for preparation, examination and post-examination (and thereby relating patient-commitment to resource-commitment), and the effective data. It should be noted that this coupling provides the only specification of time for any examination - allowing full licence for different doctors to specify their own time needs for a common examination, and for similar accommodation of other human and mechanical idiosyncracies. A maximum of eight couplings are allowed per RESOURCE.

If there are any patients booked for a newly altered RESOURCE for the five days starting with the effective date of the alteration, warning is immediately given and opportunity presented to pass to the AKTB dialog. More generally, changes in the coupling stimulate overall report of the revised situation; answering 'YES' after registering the change leads immediately to a display of the pertinent weekly operating schedule, while breaking avoids it.

Dialog BON - clinic operating schedule

The final step in establishing the basic resource records for booking is the specification of operating hours. In recording and managing the operating schedules, the System accommodates the conflicting aspects of economy of a regular pattern with the need for flexibility and variation. It also, as indicated earlier, allows reservation of certain times for urgent cases. For any one RESOURCE, the possibility of up to eight different values of EXAM being coupled adds complication to the timetable, to which the urgent lines add in effect a ninth, all-purpose, category.

The opening message of BON is of the style
BON RESOURCE date
and results in a display like that illustrated in Fig 8-15, the date entered being interpreted as indicating the week that included it, and the display showing, at this initial response stage, merely which days are operating days and which are not.

```
--------------------------------------------------------------------------
--                                                                      --
-- BON 2410 760325 OVERVIEW CLINIC OPRTG SCHED  2410 SMITH DEPT 246     --
--                                                                      --
--          ENTER DATA, LINE NR OR BREAK           r               r    --
-- APPLICABLE SCHEDULE FROM 760321                                      --
-- AUR=A  DAY                                                           --
--    .  1 MON  CLINIC                                                  --
--    .  2 TUE  CLINIC                                                  --
--    .  3 WED  NO CLINIC                                               --
--    .  4 THU  NO CLINIC                                               --
--    .  5 FRI  NO CLINIC                                               --
--                                                                      --
-- MORE SCHEDULES ARE RECORDED, NEXT APPLIES FROM 760405                --
-- NEW  SCHEDULE APPLIES FROM ...... 1   ALTERED DAY NR .               --
--                                                                      --
--                                                                      --
-- IF NEXT OVERVIEW DESIRED ANSWER YES r..                              --
--                                                                      --
--------------------------------------------------------------------------
```

FIG 8-15 BON - INITIAL RESPONSE.

The example shown advises that more schedules are recorded for succeeding periods (technically, at least one more), and gives the date at which the currently displayed schedule is superseded. If the user wishes to step on to that next schedule, it suffices to give the indicated answer 'YES' in the last line; it might be noted that the start-of-message symbol is already placed ahead of this unusual answer zone, as well as ahead of the normal one and also at the end of row 5 (instead of the more usual row 3) to cover the return transmission of the central array.

Return transmission with 'D' = Delete opposite any clinic day (i.e. in the first column), is the step toward removing all current scheduled times for that day. This process can be applied simultaneously to two or more days, and allows either complete removal of a day from the continuing schedule or a wiping clean of the slate before recreating a complicatedly different schedule.

The third alternative type of answer to such a response as Fig 8-15 is transmission of a line number, in the normal zone in row 3. This results in a detailed display for the day indicated, which is illustrated in Fig 8-16. The central array here shows, for each pertinent EXAM and equally for the all-purpose priority code ('PRTY'), the time intervals scheduled. It should be noted that the intervals are not mutually exclusive; however, overlap implies an ability to accommodate either service to the exclusion, during the actual appointment, of the other, and not an ability for parallel service.

```
¬¬¬¬¬¬¬¬¬¬¬¬¬¬¬¬¬¬¬¬¬¬¬¬¬¬¬¬¬¬¬¬¬¬¬¬¬¬¬¬¬¬¬¬¬¬¬¬¬¬¬¬¬¬¬¬¬¬¬¬¬¬¬¬¬¬¬¬¬¬¬¬
¬¬                                                                  ¬¬
¬¬ BON 2410 760325 SCHEDULE FOR 2410 SMITH DEPT 246 FROM 760325     ¬¬
¬¬ ENTER DATA, V=OVERVIEW, DAY NR OR BREAK        r               r ¬¬
¬¬ MONDAY                  ALTER DATE ......                        ¬¬
¬¬   PRIORITY TO BE RELEASED .. DAYS BEFORE EXAMINATION             ¬¬
¬¬  EXAM    FROM-TO   FROM-TO   FROM-TO   FROM-TO   FROM-TO         ¬¬
¬¬  PRTY    1000-1045 1400-1430 ....-.... ....-.... ....-....       ¬¬
¬¬  2402    700.-800. 1045-1200 1430-1600 ....-.... ....-....       ¬¬
¬¬  3320    800.-1000. 1045-1200 ....-.... ....-.... ....-....      ¬¬
¬¬                                                                  ¬¬
¬¬                                                                  ¬¬
¬¬                                                                  ¬¬
¬¬                                                                  ¬¬
¬¬                                                                  ¬¬
¬¬                                                                  ¬¬
¬¬ R= PERIOD SUBJECT TO RELEASE                                     ¬¬
¬¬ STATE YES IF RELEASE SCHEME DESIRED%..                           ¬¬
¬¬                                                                  ¬¬
¬¬¬¬¬¬¬¬¬¬¬¬¬¬¬¬¬¬¬¬¬¬¬¬¬¬¬¬¬¬¬¬¬¬¬¬¬¬¬¬¬¬¬¬¬¬¬¬¬¬¬¬¬¬¬¬¬¬¬¬¬¬¬¬¬¬¬¬¬¬¬¬
```

FIG 8-16 BON - DETAILED SCHEDULE FOR A DAY.

The reservation of any time for priority patients can result in unused appointment time if insufficient such patients eventuate. To ameliorate this if desired, any priority interval can be designated as to be released at a preset number of days prior to its occurrence. Such an interval is indicated by an 'F' instead of an '-' in the display of clock times, and the interval is specifiable above. The details of the release scheme can be pursued by giving the indicated 'YES' answer in row 16.

Answering with a day number brings the like display for the day cited, while answering after any such display with 'W' returns the overview of the week. Any alteration to the schedule requires firstly an indicating message using the overview display. If the days of operation are left unchanged (and themselves are not sufficiently changed within to justify the initial cancellation), the penultimate visible row at least must have the effective date for the change entered, plus the day number of the first day of the week for which new times are to be entered. This leads to the detailed display and the scope for establishing new times. On completion of one day, the number of the next day to be altered is given as answer, and so the process proceeds.

TRAFFIC LOAD

Because of its limited implementation, the booking sub-system contributes barely 5% of typical daily dialog traffic. However, as Table 5-1 shows, the characters communicated per dialog are distinctly above average for the System, and the impact within the computer is generally more than double that of the average dialog - reflecting the complexity of the booking process as implemented. Table 8-1 shows the relative contribution of the BOKA and BOKU dialogs, where it can be seen that the former is roughly five times the average as regards computer load per dialog. It is, in fact, the most expensive dialog outside the laboratory sub-system.

DIALOG	AVERAGE IMPACT PER DIALOG						DAILY TRAFFIC		
	TELECOMS		OTHER I/O		PROG	CPU			
	MSGS	CHARS	ACC	KWDS	CALLS	SECS	MIN	MEAN	MAX
BOKA	8	2765	124	43	35	2.20	175	269	340
BOKU	3	486	18	7	1	.20	305	424	656
ETC									
OVERALL	5	1400	58	22	12	.94	644	852	1145

TABLE 8-1 REAL-TIME PROCESSING STATISTICS FOR BOOKING SUB-SYSTEM, BASED ON TRAFFIC SURVEY 1 THRU 5 SEP 75.

(SEE TABLE 5-1 FOR EXPLANATIONS.)

CHAPTER 9

THE OUTPATIENT SUB-SYSTEM

Introduction

The outpatient sub-system was designed to collect the more salient medical and service items from among the masses of data arising from the outpatient activities of the hospitals and other medical-care facilities in the County. Since, as explained earlier, these outpatients operations cover office visits to family and specialist practitioners as much as the visits to technical departments of hospitals, the information to be gleaned provides a major part of the patient's health picture but is extremely voluminous when taken over the 1.5 million people continuously.

Besides the incidence of each visit, the sub-system includes diagnoses, operations and other procedures among the data collected. Certain specific drug regimes are recorded (insulin, anticoagulants, cortisone), and the main drug employed. With a view to study of effectiveness, provision is made for recording the result of therapy in terms of improved/unchanged/worse. Data on the referring service and the disposition of the care are also accommodated.

The outpatient subsystem was built as an associate of the booking system, intended to take over information already recorded during the booking process. However, the occurrence of unscheduled visits alone prohibits a complete dependence on the booking subsystem, and in fact the outpatient subsystem was designed without even a bias towards its associate. The patient connection of the two is via the HP and SL records of the P.R., which they, among others, share. Thus, at least personal data can pass automatically from booking to subsequent record, although much of this would be made common by the H.R. in any case. The OV record of the P.R. is unique to the outpatient sub-system, as the DBP is to the booking sub-system.

The data collected by the sub-system will normally be recorded first on paper by the doctor; as is common in the System, data entry using terminals is established as a task apart from the treatment situation. The paper record when completed or, if diagnoses are still pending, even while incomplete, is used by a medical secretary as the source document for entry through the terminal. Except for correction, completion with subsequent diagnoses, and possible reference (e.g. relative to subsequent visit), the real-time activity is predominantly the basic entry of this visit-record.

Except for the incidental collection of telephone numbers and the potential collection of vaccination and critical medical data, the outpatient sub-system has, currently, no influence on the H.R. And because of its expense in terms of storage and processing time, the sub-system is currently restricted to the one, albeit large, hospital of Huddinge.

Outpatients is the one area of health care where there is routinely a charge to patients, as well as a charge to the State Insurance Office, and the sub-system is intended to feed pertinent batch routines for the requisite accounting and billing. However, this is not currently done.

THE INPUT PROCESSES

Dialog OPVM - Recording of medical outpatient data

Transmission of
OPVM PNR/RNR DEPT
produces the form-display shown in Fig 9-1.

```
-------------------------------------------------------------------------
--                                                                     --
-- OPVM 180312+1233 403                                                --
-- RECORDING OF MEDICAL OUTPATNT DATA                                  --
-- ENTER DATA OR BREAK                              r               r --
-- PNR/RNR   180312+1233  NAME ANDERSON, ERIK CARL ROLF                --
-- TEL       ...........  NAT .. SEX M        OCCP  JOINER             --
-- ADR  33 CHESTNUT AV.............PONR 11744  PA TABY..........       --
--                                                                     --
-- VDATE  760207          VTYP .       UNSCH  .   LOCN     .. DOC .. --
-- REF FR  ..... ...      IO   .       SICKN  .   F-T  ..... .....    --
-- D1  ..... PRI ....     D2   .....   PR2   ....   D CON    D NO .   --
-- OPNC .... ANEC ....    V/S1  ..     V/S2  ..     V/S3  ..           --
-- INSLN  .  ANCOAG  .    CORT  .      DRUGC    .......                --
-- RESULT .               TO RETURN .  TRANSFER TO  .  ..... ...       --
--                                                                     --
--                                                                     --
--                                                                     --
--                                                                     --
-------------------------------------------------------------------------
```

FIG 9-1 OPVM - INITIAL COMPUTER RESPONSE.

As usual, any pertinent information on the cited patient that is already recorded in the P.R. or H.R. is included automatically in the response, while the current date is inserted as the presumed visit date (VDATE). These proffered entries must be checked, and altered as necessary, as well as the numerous further entries made. These are

- VTYP to show whether an initial, return or indirect visit
- UNSCH to show whether visit was unscheduled or not
- LOCN allows recording of location within serving department
- DOC to show attending doctor (code within department)
- REF FR allows recording of INSTN and DEPT that referred patient
- IO allows recording of whether reference was from in- or out-patient service
- SICKN provides for recording that a 'sicknote' was provided
- F-T provides for 'from' and 'to' dates of any sicknote
- D1, D2 provide for up to two diagnoses (DIAGC)
- PR1, PR2 provide for up to two procedures (local code)
- D CON provides for recording that diagnosis is under consideration
- D NO provides for positive recording that no diagnosis is to be given
- OPNC provides for operation (OPNC)
- ANEC provides for anesthetic (ANEC)
- V/S1, V/S2, V/S3 allow for vaccination and serological procedures (codes not currently established)
- INSLN, ANCOAG, CORT allow, through entry of Y=YES, recording of insulin, anticoagulant and cortisone treatment

DRUGC allows recording of one drug (<u>DRUGC</u>),

RESULT, which relates particularly to therapeutic visits, allows recording of whether the patient was thereby improved, unchanged or worse (values 1, 2 & 3 respectively).

TO RETURN, TRANSFER TO allow recording of the disposition of the patient, the latter providing for a transfer code (1 = own inpatient, 2 = other department in same hospital, 3 = other hospital), plus <u>INSTN</u> and <u>DEPT</u> as required.

Again, "to show" indicates obligatory entry; in addition to those so marked, either PR1 or DCON or DNO must be entered.

Additional diagnoses, procedures, vaccinations and operations, to a doubling of the numbers allowed here, can be recorded using the dialog OPVMF described below.

Pressing the SEND key brings the data to the usual computer checking, which can result in either an instruction to correct (or break) or to register (or alter the data and resubmit, or break).

For a return visit (VTYP = 2), the diagnosis and procedure entries can be left blank initially, and the computer then enters those recorded for the last visit (to the said department), provided these do not exceed the limit of two. These in turn can be altered in an additional step prior to registration of the transaction. If the diagnoses or procedures recorded exceed two, the fields are not filled automatically, and a warning of the excess is given at the bottom of the screen. To ascertain these entries, resort must be made to the OPVMV dialog. This ancillary dialog can be entered from OPVM as well as in the normal direct way, by entering its code in the answer zone and transmitting. The OPVMV is described below.

<u>Dialog OPVMK - Alteration of recorded medical outpatient data</u>

Transmission of

OPVMK <u>PNR</u>/<u>RNR</u> <u>DEPT</u> date

brings to the screen, in the form described for OPVM, the data recorded for the patient visit to the department and on the date specified (if any), and allows alteration of that data.

Besides the new dialog name in row 2, the display is different by the insertion of a row of data concerning the current sequence of attendance. This appears immediately below the address now, and shows the dates of the first and latest visit, plus the total number of return visits.

Except for the identifying fields of PNR/RNR, DEPT and VDATE, any of the fields can be altered within the constraints applicable to OPVM, and usual procedures followed for registration of the altered data. Where any alteration is made that naturally applies to subsequent visits in a sequence (e.g. alteration of UNSCH) the revised value is placed automatically in the subsequent records.

If the initiating message points to two or more visits, i.e. of the one patient to the one department on the one day, an overview is displayed instead of the details of a single visit. This overview lists the visits line-by-line, showing for each, as well as a line number, the VTYP and the first diagnosis. Lacking a record of the time, it is not necessarily easy to distinguish multiple visits; however, it is not likely that there be so many as to render repeated effort unacceptable. Given the overview, selection is made by answering with the line number in the standard answer zone.

Dialog OPVMF - Recording extra outpatient diagnoses

The recording of additional diagnoses to the two allowed by the OPVM, and of additional procedures, vaccinations and operations - to a total twice that allowed by the OPVM - is achieved using the OPVMF dialog. Transmission of

OPVMF PNR/RNR DEPT date

(which can be executed at the completion of the corresponding OPVM dialog by inserting the additional F of the dialog code and appending the date to the extant row 1) brings a display, in OPVM-layout, of data recorded for the cited patient, department and date. However, the fields for which additional values can be entered are left blank (and their field names adjusted to be D3, AT3, etc.,). Appropriate entries are then made in one or more of these blanks and the procedure for registration followed. Besides checking these new entries, the program checks that none of the other fields have been altered, such action being indicative of confusion as to the effect of the OPVMF dialog.

```
OPVMV 180312+1233 403
DIAGNOSES & PROCEDURES RECORDED BY OUTPATNT SERVICE
GIVE F, B OR BREAK



                     VISIT   VDATE   DIAGNOSIS  PROC
CARE PERIOD  1         C              2345
                       4    750827    1121       5656
                                      2345       2913
                       5    750831    1121       5656
                                      2345       2913
                                                 2915
                       6    750903    1121       5656
                                                 2913
                                            rF   rB   rBR CONT    r
```

FIG 9-2 OPVMV - OVERVIEW DISPLAY.

Dialog OPVMV - overview of diagnoses and procedures

The OPVMV dialog, initiated for a specific patient and department, provides a listing of the diagnoses and procedures recorded for a sequence of visits. This response is illustrated in Fig 9-2, for a continuation section of a list that exceeds the capacity of the screen, and would only be visible after use of the NEXT-PAGE feature.

This display illustrates an alternative approach for answers of having each alternative shown alongside a start-of-message symbol, so it suffices to move the cursor to the first space following the desired answer, and press SEND. However, as explained in Chapter 5, two of the illustrated answers are now on function keys.

Dialog OPVMU - retrieval of outpatient medical data

This dialog functions in essentially the same manner as OPVMK, except that it precludes alteration. As with OPVMK, the existence of more than one screenful for the specified date results in display of an overview.

Dialog OPVMO - overview of patient attendance at hospital

This dialog is more general than the foregoing by covering all departments at the pertinent hospital. Thus it is initiated by only

OPVMO PNR/RNR

and results in cursory citation of all outpatient visits within the relevant institution, as illustrated in Fig 9-3.

```
OPVMO 180312+1233
VISITS RECORDED IN OUTPATIENTS

PNR/RNR    180312+1233  NAME ANDERSON, CARL ERIK ROLF

NR   VDATE        DEPT
 1   760207        101
 2   760212        301
```

FIG 9-3 OPVMO - RESPONSE.

Dialog OPVP - recording of personal data

While OPVM and OPVMK provide for insertion and altering of personal data along with medical, the OPVP dialog is restricted to the personal data. For the patient cited, it allows insertion or alteration of any of the data fields (other than PNR/RNR) occupying rows 4 thru 6 of the OPVM display (Fig 9-1). The OPVP display has the same layout, but truncated after row 6.

FILE RELATIONSHIPS

The input processes described all relate to the construction of the OV record of the P.R. plus, as necessary, the SL record and, where initially absent, the head record of the P.R.

Telephone numbers obtained for the VL record pass routinely to the KRM record of the H.R. during the periodic batch process. Any vaccinations or critical medical diseases reported can also pass likewise to the KRM. Otherwise the outpatient data will, after the 90-day retention period on the P.R., pass to the off-line archival storage.

As with the other sub-systems the outpatient sub-system calls on the H.R. for basic personal information on newly presenting patients that are residents.

TRAFFIC LOAD

The outpatient sub-system contributes directly close to a thousand dialogs to the typical daily load, with over half being OPVM and a third being OPVMO. Table 9-1 gives the more important data concerning this traffic. As Table 5-1 shows, except for a slightly higher number of characters, the average outpatient dialog is less demanding of system resources than the overall average.

DIALOG	AVERAGE IMPACT PER DIALOG						DAILY TRAFFIC		
	TELECOMS		OTHER I/O		PROG	CPU			
	MSGS	CHARS	ACC	KWDS	CALLS	SECS	MIN	MEAN	MAX
OPVM	5	1698	21	17	7	.43	320	486	732
OPVMO	2	288	5	3	1	.07	223	299	340
ETC									
OVERALL	4	1116	14	11	4	.28	748	868	1108

TABLE 9-1 REAL-TIME PROCESSING STATISTICS FOR OUTPATIENT SUB-SYSTEM, BASED ON SURVEY OF 1 THRU 5 SEP 75.

(SEE TABLE 5-1 FOR EXPLANATIONS.)

CHAPTER 10

THE CHEMICAL LABORATORY SUB-SYSTEM

While a complete sub-system for the laboratory should cover all processes from requisitioning of the service through assembling of the individual results to reporting back to the requisitioner, the sub-system in use up to 1976 did not include any assembling of the individual results. It covered on the one hand the processes up to the point of analysis by the technician, then resumed at the point where the technician had determined the clinical values. The initial processes extend in computer form to the nursing stations, allowing staff there to enter requisitions directly into the computer records (though in practice most requisitions reach the laboratory in paper form, to be entered into the computer there). Collection and work lists then become available to laboratory staff. The later processes resume with the keying-in of the various results, including results obtained by automatic laboratory equipment, and proceeds through the production of appropriate results reports - with on-line enquiry access being simultaneously available to nursing staffs.

A process flow diagram is provided as Fig 10-1. At the top of the diagram is the BPA dialog, which provides for the requisitioning of tests by a patient-serving unit. This could be an inpatient or outpatient nursing unit but in practice is invariably the central patient laboratory. The lines immediately following show the normal practice for nursing units, with the requisitions being entered into the computer by laboratory clinical staff, using the RAS & RAS5 dialogs. The manual sorting process here is on a location basis and is aimed at facilitating entry - in particular, allowing specimen numbers to be assigned before entry.

Overnight processing at Datacentral produces both collection lists and laboratory work lists in preparation for the early morning collection rounds and the subsequent technical work. While this latter proceeds, additional requisitions are continuously acceptable at Datacentral; these are incorporated into the work programme via the PAM dialog.

Following analysis, the results are entered into the computer using RES, RUS or BUS (and commented upon using KOR). Concurrently the nursing units can enter, using REP, any urinalysis results they obtain using the simple stick test. Access to these various results is then obtainable with the POL, OAR & NYS dialogs - the first for laboratory staff and the others for different needs of nursing staff. Printed confirmation of the results, together with various laboratory management reports, occurs during the succeeding night.

The test codes used represent variously individual tests, machine groupings of tests and standard batteries of tests.

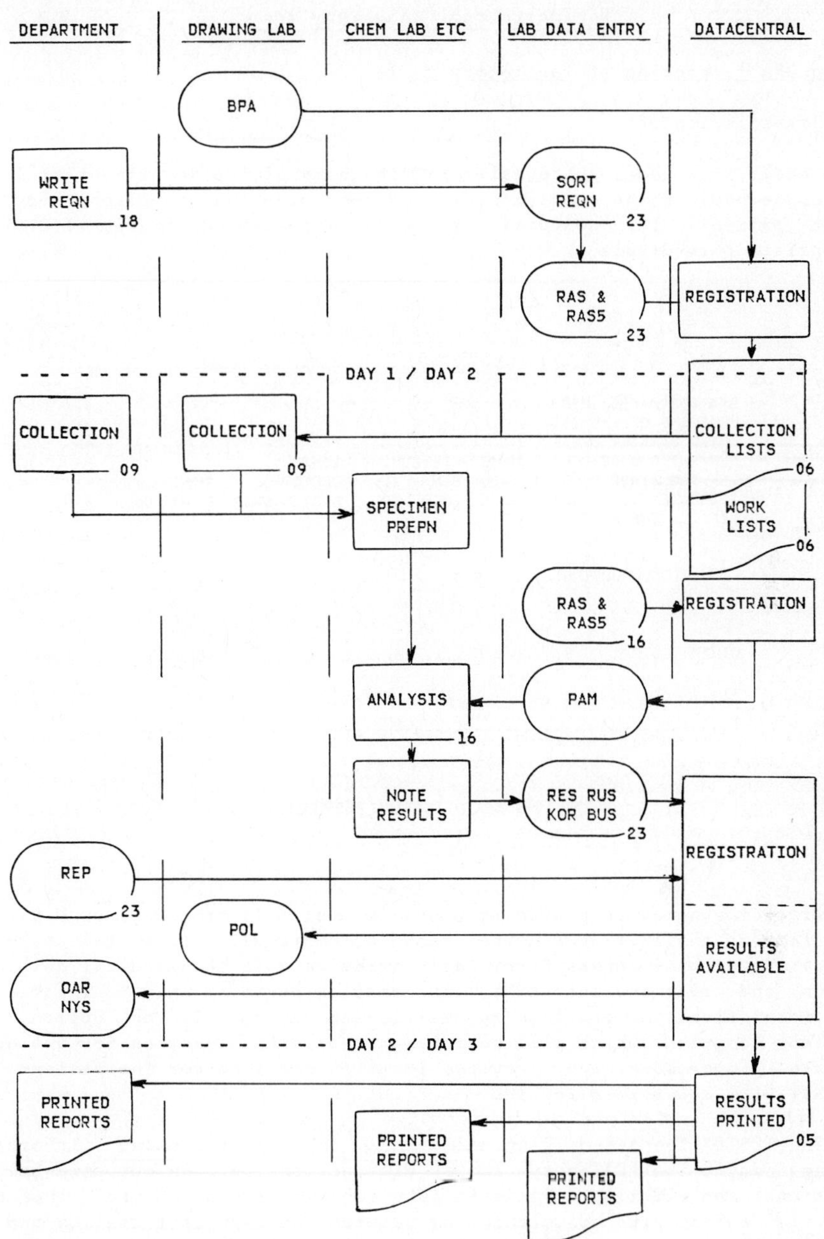

FIG 10-1 OVERALL FLOW IN LAB SUB-SYSTEM

SUFFIX NUMBERS INDICATE HOUR FOR COMPLETION.

ARRANGING FOR LABORATORY TESTS

Dialog BPA - ordering of laboratory test

Transmission of
BPA PNR/RNR abcde
where abcde is a local abbreviation of the name of the department or lesser unit concerned, is the initial step in direct ordering of a laboratory test for a patient. The computer response, illustrated in Fig 10-2, is an appropriate form-display.

```
-------------------------------------------------------------------
--                                                                --
-- BPA 00202+0063 MED                                             --
-- ORDERING OF LAB TEST                                           --
-- ENTER DATA OR BREAK                                            --
-- PNR/RNR 000202+0063   NAME PETERSON, PAULINA                   --
-- REF INS 11002     DEPT ...    STN   ...   DOCTOR ..    RM&B  .... --
-- SPECDATE ......   CAT  ..     LOCN  CPL   BKGTIM 0000  RTIM  0000 --
-- HEP .   INF N                                                  --
--  .                .                     .                      --
--  .                .                     .                      --
--  .   BLOODGROUPING  .   ECG             .                      --
--                                                                --
--                                                                --
--                                                                --
-- OTHER TESTS       B ....   B ....  B ....   B ....    B ....   --
--                                                                --
--                                                                --
--                                                                --
-------------------------------------------------------------------
```

FIG 10-2 BPA - INITIAL RESPONSE.

After the name, displayed as usual if available from P.R. or H.R., and the referring institution's number known automatically from the terminal record, the display covers first administrative data then medical data. The station and room-and-bed (RM&B) information pertains only to inpatients, while identification of the requisitioning doctor is an option. The inpatient location, which will be interpreted as the location for taking of specimen, supersedes any previous location recorded for the patient with the chemistry sub-system records.

The TESTDATE entered is normally that of the following (laboratory working) day. The CATegory is a distinction between outpatients, new admissions, and existing inpatients. The location indicated for the next field is merely the discriminator between the inpatient station and the Central Patient Laboratory; since the BPA dialog is used predominantly for the latter and its outpatient clientele, the computer makes the presumptive entry. The next fields allow for recording of any time commitments, one for taking of the specimen and the next for provision of result; the latter is not currently in operation. Before proceeding to specification of tests to be carried out, provision is made for recording, through entry of Y = Yes, any known risk of hepatitis or of other infection that pertains; the latter field has a presumptive N = No already entered.

The test specification area comprises nine specific locations plus five general ones, the former covering the more commonly requested tests - identified by textual names - and the latter allowing the entry of standard test codes. In specifying any test, the entry is normally R = required, but the alternative T = telephoned can be inserted if urgency warrants having the laboratory telephone the result as soon as it is available. The routine entry is already placed alongside the code fields of the miscellaneous tests, where entry of a code means selection, but each occurrence can be overwritten as appropriate. The nine identified tests are

Dialogs RAS & RAS5 - recording of tests and specimen numbers

While the BPA group of dialogs is oriented to the intermittent requisitioning of tests by a patient-serving unit - albeit the Central Patient Laboratory usually - the RAS group is oriented to the entry of requisitions by the main laboratory office, at a processing point where specimen numbers can be established. As shown in Fig 10-1, this situation is reached after submission of requisition forms to the laboratory department, and is preceded by a sorting of the forms into an order convenient to the laboratory.

```
RAS   475 760212
RECORDING OF TESTS AND SPECIMEN NUMBERS 760212      INSTN  11002
ENTER DATA OR BREAK
 SPEC-NR  PERSON-NUMB  H URG   INSTN  DEPT STN  DOC  K P  STIM
 12- 475  ......-....  . ....  .....  ...  ...  ..   . .  ....

   ....   ....   ....   ....   ....
   ....   ....   ....   ....   ....
   ....   ....   ....   ....   ....
   ....   ....   ....   ....   ....
```

FIG 10-3 RAS - INITIAL RESPONSE.

Both RAS and RAS5 involve entry of a specimen number along with the requisition details for each patient, and rely entirely on the entry of test code numbers rather than the distinctive display of selected common tests; their key difference lies in RAS being for a single patient per dialog and RAS5 being for several, in fact up to five. Figs 10-3 and 10-4 illustrate their similarities and differences at the initial response stage.

In both illustrations, the top row shows an initiating message that includes a number and a date. The former is the specimen number for the patient, or first patient, to be entered with the dialog, and the date is

```
--------------------------------------------------------------------
--                                                                --
-- RAS5  475 760212                                               --
-- RECORDING OF TESTS AND SPECIMEN NUMBERS                        --
-- ENTER DATA OR BREAK                                            --
-- SPEC-NR  PERSON-NUMB  KSH INSTN  DEPT STN  DOC TESTC TESTC TESTC --
-- 12- 475  ......-....  ... 11002  ...  ...  ..  ....  ....  .... --
-- ....                                           ....  ....  .... --
-- 12- 476  ......-....  ... 11002  ...  ...  ..  ....  ....  .... --
-- ....                                           ....  ....  .... --
-- 12- 477  ......-....  ... 11002  ...  ...  ..  ....  ....  .... --
-- ....                                           ....  ....  .... --
-- 12- 478  ......-....  ... 11002  ...  ...  ..  ....  ....  .... --
-- ....                                           ....  ....  .... --
-- 12- 479  ......-....  ... 11002  ...  ...  ..  ....  ....  .... --
-- ....                                                           --
--                                                                --
--                                                                --
--                                                                --
--------------------------------------------------------------------
```

FIG 10-4 RAS5 - INITIAL RESPONSE.

the specimen date involved (the day part of which, as can be seen, is used as the stem for the full specimen numbers). If the date is omitted from the initiating message the current date is assumed. If zero is entered as the starting specimen numbers, the computer assumes the first free number and displays it below; for the current date the zero can be omitted, leaving only the dialog code.

Most of the fields of the RAS and RAS5 are comprehensible via the BPA dialog. The CUH column of the RAS5 is actually three independent columns, the C and the H covering, as they do in RAS also, the category and hepatitis fields. The U refers to urgency, which is labelled URG in the RAS dialog and which was associated with each selection in the BPA.

Appropriate correction - RASK - and viewing - RASU & RAS5U - dialogs are provided.

Collection lists and work lists

The various requisitioned tests entered during the day by the BPA, RAS and RAS5 dialogs are assembled during the night and printed in collection-list and work-list reports for the impending day. Each of the two types includes both printouts on continuous paper and print-outs on labels, and each type is divided into separate report pages for the separate sections and staff concerned. As all hepatitis risk specimens are processed in a special laboratory, these are excluded from the normal work list for each test involved and included in special work lists. Separate work lists are prepared for each individually requisitionable test and for each test-group, and show the upper and lower bounds of the normal range for each test they cover. Below this, the requisitions are listed in order of specimen number. Patient, patient's location and priority are shown for each, following marked areas for manual recording of the result.

The additional work requirements arising during the laboratory working day are accessed using a PAM (or PAMH for hepatitis-risk specimens) dialog, citing the test-code concerned. Although the response is a list of specimens on the screen, a printed copy is immediately available via the associated slave printer. This list identifies the patient and nursing unit alongside each specimen number.

RECORDING THE RESULTS

Dialog RES - recording of results by specimen number

This dialog provides the means for entry of the test results obtained in relation to the work lists. The initial response of the computer to an initiating message is a form-display similar to the incomplete part of the work list, together with sufficient identifying data. Identification relates to two variables - the tests performed and the specimens involved. Hence the initiating message must indicate the values of each concerned. For the test(s), the normal test code is entered after the dialog code. Then follows the identification of the first specimen involved. Since the purpose is to enter results for specimen tests lacking results, specimens already having results are ignored by the RES dialog. Hence in fact the specimen number entered merely represents the starting point for extraction of uncompleted cases. As before, lack of date is taken to imply the current date, and zero or lack of any entry after the test code is taken to mean starting at the beginning. Examples of the initiating message are

    RES 100 16 760120

meaning test (group) code 100, starting with the first incompleted example after specimen 16 of the cited date,

    RES 1001

meaning test code 1001, starting with the first uncompleted specimen, of the current day

    RES 1001 6

meaning test code 1001, starting with the first uncompleted specimen after number 6 of today.

The form-display that appears in response varies in layout not only according to the test code, but also according to whether the code represents a single- or multiple-result procedure. Figs 10-5 and 10-6 give examples of the respective layouts, where it can be observed that the singular case provides for several specimens to a row while the multiple case uses a row for one specimen. The simpler case also provides the upper and lower normal values in its display. As can be seen, the standard provision for each answer is five characters. The style allowable depends on the specification of the test - the range being described under DIM in Appendix C. However, as noted there, certain alphabetic results are allowable for any test in order to record failure or inadequacy of the material. Besides the routine interpretation of the dialog code, both the test code and the date (explictly or implicitly entered) are translated into their textual equivalents, the latter being as day of the week.

Besides marking unacceptable entries with an F = Fail during data checking, the computer marks exceptional values with

- * if outside normal range but within experienced range
- ? if outside experienced range - this being accompanied by a general message, set to flash, in row 15.

If there is a further incomplete specimen in the group, the registration process is followed by an invitation to enter next specimen number and transmit.

```
--------------------------------------------------------------------------
--                                                                      --
-- RES       1001      0      760120                                    --
-- RECORDING OF RESULTS BY SPEC-NR FOR TEST B-SR                        --
-- ENTER DATA OR BREAK                                                  --
-- SPECDATE 760120                     NORMAL LIMITS 2     -11          --
--    SNR  RESLT        SNR  RESLT      SNR  RESLT       SNR  RESLT     --
--     13  .....         18  .....       21  .....        24  .....     --
--     25  .....         31  .....       48  .....        49  .....     --
--     50  .....         52  .....       58  .....        62  .....     --
--     67  .....         68  .....       70  .....        76  .....     --
--     84  .....         94  .....       98  .....       102  ....      --
--    103  .....        104  .....      105  .....       108  .....     --
--                                                                      --
--                                                                      --
--                                                                      --
--                                                                      --
--                                                                      --
--                                                                      --
--------------------------------------------------------------------------
```

FIG 10-5 RES - INITIAL RESPONSE FOR SINGLE-RESULT TEST

```
--------------------------------------------------------------------------
--                                                                      --
-- RES       100      0      760120                                     --
-- RECORDING OF RESULTS BY SPEC-NR FOR TEST B-ROUTINE BLOOD STATUS      --
-- ENTER DATA OR BREAK                                                  --
-- SPECDATE 760120                                                      --
--    SNR  WHITE     RED       HB      HCT      MCV     MCH     MCHC    --
--     11  X....     X....     .....   .....    X....   X....   X....   --
--     22  X....     X....     .....   .....    X....   X....   X....   --
--     43  X....     X....     .....   .....    X....   X....   X....   --
--     77  X....     X....     .....   .....    X....   X....   X....   --
--     80  X....     X....     .....   .....    X....   X....   X....   --
--     81  X....     X....     .....   .....    X....   X....   X....   --
--                                                                      --
--                                                                      --
--                                                                      --
--                                                                      --
--                                                                      --
--                                                                      --
--------------------------------------------------------------------------
```

FIG 10-6 RES - INITIAL RESPONSE FOR MULTI-RESULT TEST

Dialog RESK - correction following RES dialog

For a limited time after entry, the results recorded via the RES dialog can be altered using the RESK dialog. The initial procedure is similar to that for RES, but with the provision that a specimen number must be entered. The resulting response is likewise similar except that it covers just the one specimen and shows the currently recorded value(s). Correction is then a matter of keying in the changes and proceeding as with a RES dialog.

Dialog RESU - observing data recorded via RES/RESK

The RESU provides the same multi-specimen coverage as the RES, and effectively re-displays the final RES screen for the specimens identified, but with any RESK alterations effected. The zero/blank specimen identification can be used in the initiating message; whatever the specification, all specimens from that one are displayed, with blank in the results field where appropriate. The visual qualification of exceptional values is retained.

Dialog RUS - composite requisition and results.

To avoid, for urgent and other special cases, both the laboriousness of successive entry and the complications of having to await entry of requisition before entering results, a composite requisition/results dialog is provided in the form of RUS. The basic entry is RUS followed by a test-code, but this may be followed by a specimen number and also a date. Any entered specimen number is taken only as a proffered one by the computer, to be used only if it is not currently free; otherwise the next free number is assigned. The consequential form-display provides a line for identification of the usual requisition details then identified fields for the one to 36 results implied as occurring by the test-code entered.

No special correction or viewing dialogs are provided in association with RUS; RASK, RASU, RESK, etc., are effective.

Dialogs BUS & BUSK - additional tests and results.

Where laboratory results indicate an immediate need for additional tests on an existing specimen (or other equivalent reason exists), an existing requisition can be augmented by direct insertion of the additional results using the BUS dialog. This functions similarly to RUS, except that an existing specimen number must be entered, and the line of patient data is provided automatically. The associated dialog BUSK provides for related correction, and includes in its form-display response all requisitioned tests (up to the maximum of 36 feasible). Conversely, any tests added via BUS are viewable along with others through the RASU dialog.

Dialogs KOR & KORP - commenting on results.

All of the above dialogs for entry of results relate to compact results, and offer no latitude for elaboration, verbal qualification or other comment. The dialog KOR fulfills this need, allowing the entry of up to 40 text-free characters for any one requisitioned test. Once again the opening message follows the dialog code with the test-code, which must then be followed by the specimen number and, if other than the current day's, the date concerned. The response is illustrated in Fig 10-7; it includes identifying data, the result recorded for the test, and any comment already recorded. Besides licence to change the 40-character comment field, thereby entering an initial comment or amending to any degree an existing one, the compact result is equally open to alteration within this dialog. Hence it functions as an alternative to RESK and BUSK, but specifically for one test at a time. Those others are executable only relevant to specimens of current day or the preceding day. With KOR corrections can be applied to older specimens, but this in turn is limited to one month. For still older specimens the dialog KORP must be used to effect any corrections; it

```
--------------------------------------------------------------------------
--                                                                      --
-- KOR  5539  205   751101                                              --
-- COMMENTING ON AND CORRECTING RESULTS                                 --
-- GIVE COMMENT, CORRECT RESULT OR BREAK                                --
--                                                                      --
-- PNR:  000101+0073   NAME: PETERSON, PETER JAMES                      --
-- REF:  INS: 11002    DEPT: 101      STN:  K66      DOC:  0   CAT: I   --
--                                                                      --
-- SPEC-NR:  1- 205    SDATE: 751101 STIME: 1200      PRTY:-            --
--                                                                      --
-- TEST: 5539   U-GLUCOSE                                 REF-VALU 0-0  --
-- RESULT:                                                              --
-- COMMENT:   SPECIMEN TAKEN. RESULT TOMORROW                           --
--                                                                      --
--                                                                      --
--                                                                      --
--                                                                      --
--                                                                      --
--------------------------------------------------------------------------
```

FIG 10-7 KOR - INITIAL RESPONSE

requires the additional safeguard of having PNR/RNR entered initially, but functions otherwise identically to KOR.

Dialog REP - entry of result by PNR/RNR.

As described in the introduction to the sub-system, provision is made for entry to the laboratory record of some simple tests carried out by nursing staff at the care unit. Since no specimen number is involved, identification is by PNR/RNR then date then time. (Time can be omitted, but any duplication within the one date will cause overwriting if no discrimination is provided by time.) Only six test-codes are accommodated by REP, and these are represented by six columns on the pertinent displays. A first column identifies the patient, up to six being accommodable; date and time must be the same for all patients and tests covered by one dialog.

The six tests accommodated cover pH, protein, glucose, ketone, bilirubin and blood in urine; except for a numerical pH the results recordable by this means are purely positive/negative.

PUBLISHING THE RESULTS

Laboratory results must be available promptly to allow their use in patient care, but must also be available in organized printed form to meet operational and legal requirements relative to the medical record. The System provides both an immediate accessibility via terminals to any results entered into the computer and routine printing out of the various results for each patient.

Dialog OAR - viewing the results in general.

The entry of
OAR PNR/RNR

provides immediate display of all results currently available for the patient cited, or at least all that will fit on the screen - with the newest being first. Fig 10-8 illustrates a response, and shows that, besides identifying specimen date and test then giving the result, the normal range is shown and results outside it are asterisked. If coagulation, haemolysis or such precluded a proper result, an appropriate abbreviation appears in the result column. A 'YES' under the heading 'CMNT' indicates the existence of a comment; this can be viewed by entering the relevant line number in the answer zone and transmitting, the response to which is similar to that for dialog KOR. Only eight results can be accommodated by a screenful, but mere pressing of the appropriate key or pair of keys brings automatic 'page-turning'.

```
OAR 190404+0167
OVERVIEW OF TESTS AND RESULTS
ENTER F FOR FORWARD, B FOR BACK< LNR OR BREAK
 PNR
 LNR  SDATE   STIME TEST                 RES   COMM  NORM-VALU
   1  751106  0000  U-GLUCOSE            NEG          NEG-NEG
   2  751106  0000  U-KETONES            NEG          NEG-NEG
   3  751106  0000  U-GLUCOSE              .5*          0.0
   4  751101  0900  B-WHITE CELLS         3.0         3.0-9.0
   5  751101  0900  B-RED CELLS           3.4         3.4-5.5
   6  751101  0900  B-HB                  110         110-160
   7  751101  0900  B-MCV                  75          75-100
   8  751101  0900  U-GLUCOSE            +    *       NEG-NEG
CONTD
```

FIG 10-8 OAR - INITIAL RESPONSE

Clearly the limited screen capacity usually precludes simultaneous display of successive results for one test-code; often it means that a page-turn must be executed to see even the current day's result for some test-code. To obviate such problems, and more generally remove extraneous material, the opening message can be elaborated by adding a test-code after the PNR/RNR. The result is to limit the display response to just results pertinent to that code.

The test names given show prefixes 'U' = urine and 'B' = (general) blood in Fig. 10-8. Other prefixes include ones distinguishing capillary blood, venous blood, arterial blood, serum, liquor, faeces and so on.

A printed version of the display is available immediately via the associated slave printer.

Dialog NYS - viewing new results.

To facilitate access to new results concerning their patients, the dialog NYS is provided. It is oriented to station rather than patient, that is the entry message identifies a station and the results displayed are those applying to any patient on the station. However, any one dialog applies only to one test-code, which must be identified in the initiating message prior to the station; date is again a final option, for entry where the enquiry relates to specimens taken the preceding day. Fig 10-9 illustrates the display on the screen, which again is available for immediate printing.

```
------------------------------------------------------------------------
--                                                                    --
-- NYS    0107    K66   760211                                        --
-- CHEMLAB NEW RES  DEPT K66  SPECDATE: 760211   B-GLUCOSE  0700HRS --
-- HRS  PERSON-NR    NAME                              GLU07          --
-- 0700 000101+0063 PETERSON, PETER JAMES               2.7*          --
-- 0700 190404+0167 PETERSON, PUTTE                     4.5           --
-- 0700 261213+8319 SELANDER, KLAUS                    10.2*          --
--                                                                    --
-- END OF RESULTS. PRESS PRINT FOR HARD COPY                          --
-- DIALOG CLOSED                                                      --
--                                                                    --
--                                                                    --
--                                                                    --
--                                                                    --
--                                                                    --
--                                                                    --
--                                                                    --
------------------------------------------------------------------------
```

FIG 10-9 NYS - RESPONSE

Routine printed reports for each patient

Each patient for whom there has been any laboratory activity during the day is the subject of a cumulative laboratory report, printed overnight for distribution during the early morning. This report is cumulative for up to ten days - recommencing with results for a single day as each ten-day report is completed; hence both management of the patient and the legal record require more than report for any patient staying beyond 10 days.

After identifying the patient, the reporting unit, the period being covered and the admission date where pertinent, the report presents the results grouped in the following order:- general blood tests, serum tests, arterial blood tests, urine tests, faeces analyses, general patient tests, composite tests. For each test the report shows the time of specimen-taking, the name and normal range for the test, and the results. Any comments are inserted between the blocks of results, and referred to by means of alphabetical identifications that are cited against the relevant results. All new results are highlighted by exclamation marks.

Dialog POL - Patient overview for laboratory

To meet the particular needs of laboratory staff, a variation from OAR is provided in the form of the POL dialog. Again the basic usage relates to one patient, and the constituent answers are displayed in reverse chronological order. However, the initial response relates to specimens rather than tests, these latter being available only at a second stage of the dialog. Besides identifying the (reverse) successive specimens from the patient in question, the response display gives the total number of results and the total number of comments arising from each specimen. The last eight specimens are displayed initially, together with a count of the total number on record; normal 'page-turning' provides comparable access to the balance. Augmenting of the initiating message by a date will limit the specimens displayed to those of that date pertaining to the patient cited.

An additional second stage of the dialog is enterable by responding with a line number. This leads to a display of the various tests performed on the specimen so identified (which in themselves can again exceed one screenfull). Fig 10-10 illustrates this second stage response. The only

```
--------------------------------------------------------------------------
--                                                                      --
-- POL 000101+0073                                                      --
-- PATIENT OVERVIEW FOR LAB                                             --
-- ENTER T-CD FOR COMMENT, F FOR FWRD, RETURN OR BRT                    --
-- PNR:  000101+0073   NAME: PETERSON, PETER JAMES                      --
-- REF INS:   11002    DEPT: 101     STN:  K66     DOC: 12  CAT:   I    --
-- SPEC-NR:  5- 200    SDAT: 7511-5  STIME: 1200                        --
-- T-CD  TEST-NAME             RESLT   COMM    NORM-VALU   UNITS        --
-- 1030  B-WHITE BLOODCR         3.0           3.0-9.0     MIL/L        --
-- 1020  B-RED BLOODCR           3.4           3.4-5.5     BIL/L        --
-- 1010  B-HB                  COMM     YES    110-160     G/L          --
-- 1004  B-HAEMATOCRIT           55*            37-50      VOL%         --
-- 1006  B-MCV                   75             75-100     FL           --
-- 1005  B-MCH                   26             26-35      PG           --
-- CONTD                                                                --
-- 1010 COMMENT: SPECIMENT TAKEN> RESULT TOMORROW                       --
--                                                                      --
--                                                                      --
--------------------------------------------------------------------------
```

FIG 10-10 POL - DETAILED RESPONSE

information so displayed that is additional to that of OAR is the test-code values and their corresponding units of measure, plus some general requisitioning data redundant to the normal users of OAR (e.g. location and doctor). Any comment indicated is displayed in the bottom row of the screen if the user answers with the pertinent test code (there being no line numbers).

MAINTAINING THE CATALOGUE OF TESTS

The catalogue of tests upon which the applicational dialogs depend, inclusive of the various attributes pertaining to each, is itself maintained by a set of real-time dialogs operated in the normal manner. As in many other sectors, a trio of dialogs provides for the creation, alteration and viewing of records. In this case the actual codes vary in the first character, being RAP, AAP and OAP respectively.

Dialog RAP - establishing a test-code

The opening message in the establishing a new test involves entering both the test-code value and the relevant test-type code, namely

0 for a single test, not a constituent of a group
1 for a single test, constituent of a group
2 for a group of tests
3 for a standard battery

The form-display response varies according to this type because, for instance, just the latter two types require entry of their constituents while just the former two require entry of normal values. However, the latter two differ betwen themselves in that a group test has, for instance, a standard work value while the battery is purely an entry convenience.

Types 0 and 1 have essentially identical response to the initiating message, illustrated in Fig 10-11 (assuming the test-code value entered was not already in use). Following space for a test name of up to 17 characters is a field to identify the general material required (e.g. 0 = blood, 1 = urine, 2 = faeces, 3 = liquor, 6 = patient in some whole sense, as for an electrocardiogram, 7 = some mixture) then a field already entered with the value given for test-code in the initiating message. This third field accommodates five characters and provides for the definition of a brief name for the test. This is normally availed of for individual tests (e.g. 'NA+K', 'HB', 'UREA', 'UPROT'), leaving groups and batteries with their test-code numerical values as names. The next field, also preset, necessarily has the value 0; its purpose is to allow subsequent relegation of a test to inactive status while maintaining its catalogue position as a means for interpreting historical records. The next field provides for an indication of the normal number of days required for completion of the test, and the last field in the first line of the array allows for a sequential status to be given to any test - allowing appropriate sequencing of two or more tests that must be done in a specific order.

Since the System applies across the County, provision is made in the test code specification for identifying the institution providing the test; following this is provision to identify the department and section (relevant to tests other than the biochemical tests inferred by the name of the sub-system, and even other than those normally included under clinical pathology). The next two fields, both pre-set to zero, allow, by insertion of a non-zero value, the identification of such exceptions as those tests carried out by nursing staff and reported by the REP dialog, and as those only requisitionable by laboratory staff as a consequential test (using dialog BUS or RUS). The succeeding pair of fields provide for recording the volume of material required and the means ofK collection. If the test relates to capillary blood and requires an associated test of venous blood, that other test is identified in the next field. Finally in this second entry line there is a field to record the number of costing units per test.

The penultimate entry line is entirely preset, all four fields relating to the inclusion of the test in various lists - the sectional list of tests, the laboratory work list, the laboratory protocols report and the test label ourput. The final entry line relates to the style and range of results. The first field specifies dimension; values 0 through 3 define positive numerical answers expressed as integers but representing the corresponding number of decimal places, others specify pos/neg, a range of colours, and so on. The next two pairs of fields provide for low and high

```
RAP  9999 0
REGISTERING A TEST-CODE TYPE 0
ENTER DATA OR BREAK
  TEST-NAME            MTRL   CODE    INACT  DAYS   SEQ    REF
  ..................   .      9999.   0      ..     ...    ....
  INS    DEPT   STN    TAKE   RESLT   VOL    SPEC   ASSC   WK-US
  .....  ...    ...    0      0       ....   ..     0...   0...
  SECN   LAB    LPRPT  LBL
  0...   L      L      L
  DIM    VAL L  VAL H  NORML  NORMH
  ..     .....  .....  .....  .....
```

FIG 10-11 RAP - INITIAL RESPONSE

ILLUSTRATED, AS INDICATED ON FIRST TWO ROWS, FOR TYPE 0; TYPE 1 IS IDENTICAL IN EVERY OTHER REGARD

practical limits then low and high normal-range limits. Finally comes a field for abbreviated textual expression of the units of measure applicable.

Where a test-group is being specified (i.e. type 2) the last line shown in Fig 10-12 is omitted, and replaced by accommodation for the entry of the test-codes included within the group. For a test-battery, this switch is more extensive, all of the fourth line and some of the third being deleted while the entry capacity for contitutent test codes is increased to four rows of nine. The codes included in a battery can be any of type 0, 1 or 2; a test-group on the other hand is limited to tests of type 1.

Whichever the type of test being added to the catalogue, these various fields are filled in and the completed form-display transmitted, at such time the appropriate checks and cross-checks are carried out prior to acceptance.

Dialog AAP - amendment of catalogued test

The amendment dialog AAP functions in all essentials just like the creative RAP dialog. Even the initiating message looks the same by including the type-code; this is not required for identification of the test under amendment but is used to assert the type-code that the test is to be - i.e. it is the means of effecting a change in type-code. Although the inclusion of an amendment within an initiating message is very unusual within the System, it is pertinent to include it here in this situation so as to prompt the correct form display for the task at hand. The form-display produced includes all values obtainable from the extant computer record. Since the only changes of type allowed are between 0 and 1, and between 2 and 3, the display is mostly if not totally set from the old record.

The AAP dialog is meant to serve only true amendment of an existing test, but not its wholesale revision into some other test - one reason for such limitation being the need to maintain the catalogue for historical reasons. Consequently, there are limitations to the alterations that can be effected, e.g. a quantitative test cannot have its result dimension changed to a qualitative type.

Dialog OAP - viewing the catalogued tests

Initiating an OAP dialog with an existing test-code cited results in a display of the style occurring for RAP or AAP. No type is cited in the message but the appropriate value occurs in row 2 of the display, just as with the related dialogs.

Printed reports from the catalog

Printed reports of various ordering and content are available from Datacentral. One provides a listing of all groups and batteries, listed in alphabetical order of full name and showing the constituent tests (test-code and abbreviated name) and their types. Another example provides all parameters for all tests applicable to any one specimen type (e.g. blood) The catalogue of tests is also printed periodically in a form suitable for distribution to requisitioning and other staff.

LABORATORY MANAGEMENT REPORTS

Monthly, quarterly and annual reports covering both work volumes and the experience with results are routinely prepared. Given sufficient (i.e. more than 10) results for any numerical test, the arithmetic mean and standard deviation are calculated, and displayed along with the extreme values experienced in the period and the count of results within normal range. Analyses of such facets as the numbers of urgent requisitions - by test-code, stage of the week and period with the day - are available at request.

TRAFFIC LOAD

Although providing only 10% of the dialogs, the typical dialog in the laboratory sub-system is much more extensive than the System average, in communication and computer events. As Table 5-1 shows, whereas most sub-systems are typified by 4 or 5 messages per dialog, aggregating up to 1500 characters transmitted, the laboratory sub-system averages 8 messages and over 2000 characters. The difference is still more notable within the computer, the average laboratory dialog being twice the next - that of the booking sub-system - and over four times the overall average in terms of accesses, words transferred, program calls and c.p.u. time.

Table 10-1 provides an analysis of the laboratory load, and shows RES to provide the largest overall load in the c.p.u., but RUS to have the largest unit demand in c.p.u. time as well as aggregating the most input/output in all regards.

DIALOG	AVERAGE IMPACT PER DIALOG						DAILY TRAFFIC		
	TELECOMS		OTHER I/O		PROG	CPU			
	MSGS	CHARS	ACC	KWDS	CALLS	SECS	MIN	MEAN	MAX
RES	8	2023	170	55	55	3.25	252	307	335
RUS	25	8035	516	218	99	7.33	91	119	181
OAR	5	1364	20	18	21	.48	289	392	459
RASU5	9	3591	92	34	103	1.16	12	19	32
RAS5	14	5955	478	145	71	5.74	16	38	64
BPA	7	2031	49	35	8	.75	205	294	489
BUS	13	3316	253	108	60	3.74	50	61	75
BUSK	17	3995	396	150	89	5.19	9	19	25
ETC									
OVERALL	8	2250	119	51	33	1.90	1297	1636	1844

TABLE 10-1 REAL-TIME PROCESSING STATISTICS FOR CHEM. LAB. SUB-SYSTEM, BASED ON SURVEY 1 THRU 5 SEP 75.

(SEE TABLE 5-1 FOR EXPLANATIONS.)

CHAPTER 11

BATCH PROCESSES

While the focus of this book is the real-time processes, these, as has already been seen, depend on batch processing for the entry of any person in the H.R., and in certain other regards. In fact, the H.R. is completely dependent on batch processing for its updating; in real-time processes this central file is available only for information retrieval.

Updating

Insertion in and removal from the H.R. of people is a weekly activity using data provided by the central registry office on magnetic tape. Except for file linkage and other housekeeping data, this is the sole means of altering the CFU records. The data in the medical files is updated somewhat less frequently, using both data from the P.R.s and data from outside the real-time processes. The latter route includes all the data concerning x-rays, for storage in RTG records, and virtually all the medical data that goes to the KRM records. The telephone numbers, however, as well as the inpatient-stay data, come directly from the P.R.s., except for that rapidly declining number of hospitals not converted to the inpatient sub-system.

This taking of data from the P.R.s results directly only in the changing of control flags in these files; the actual removal of the data occurs only subsequently during the periodical process - currently executed monthly on each file. In contrast to the H.R., the P.R.s are essentially real-time files, as much in the updating as in the retrieval sense. The V.R. is similarly a fully real-time file. In one small detail, however, both P.R.s and V.R. are affected by the weekly batch update of the H.R., namely through a provision whereby the departure of people from the County is signified. For a death this entails effective removal of the person from the V.R.

Routine Reports

The preparation of those various routine periodic reports, concerning numbers of admissions and so on, that are ubiquitously demanded by governmental authorities or hospital managements, is naturally a batch process that uses the P.R.s and related files. Besides the more usual reports, the Stockholm system provides extensive analyses by diagnosis. These reports are generated for two levels of diagnostic differentration - the '99-level' that covers just 99 different diagnoses groupings and the '999-level' that covers 999 finer groupings. The reports are segregated organizationally down to a sub-specialty division or clinic within a hospital, with higher-level consolidations being provided. They are produced annually, to cover one calendar year.

The 99 or 999 diagnoses itemized in any report are those that are most common for the particular specialty across the County as a whole. Thus the report for an orthopaedic surgery or ophthalmology unit at a particular hospital would be itemized only according to the most common diagnoses within the surgical field of the whole County. In the case of the '99' report, illustrated in Fig 11-1, the ranking within the sub-specialty

```
STOCKHOLM COUNTY COUNCIL            INPATIENT DISCHARGES DURING 1971
HEALTH- AND MEDICAL-CARE
CENTRAL OFFICE                      SPECIALTY      SURGERY            OPHTHAL DEPT
OPERATIONS DEPT                     SUB-SPECIALTY: OPHTHALMOLOGY      KAROLINSKA HOSPITAL
******************************************************************************************************************
 DIAG WITHIN 99-LIST     *STAY DAYS = SD      *CASES = CS   *PAT'NTS = PA*MEAN *% OF SPECLT*ADMISSION CONDN %  *+
   *  *                  *                    *             *            *DAYS *           * ACUTE *NON-ACU*NOT*-
RANK *CD*NAME            *NUMBER *  %   * CUM *NUMBER*  %   *NUMBER*  %  * OF  *SD *CS *PA *HOM*OTH*HOM*OTH*KNW* CD
SP*DP*  *                *       *      *  %  *      *      *      *     *STAY *   *   *   *                   *
******************************************************************************************************************
 1* 1*33*CATARACT        *   3145* 24.3* 24.3*   266* 11.3*   242* 13.3* 11.8* 44* 41* 39*  0*  0*  0*  0*100*-33
 2* 2*35*OTHER EYE DIS   *   2659* 20.6* 44.9*   386* 16.3*   332* 18.2*  6.9* 46* 66* 64*  1*  0*  3*  0* 96* 35
 3* 3*32*INFLAM EYE DIS  *   2257* 17.4* 62.3*   261* 11.0*   236* 13.0*  8.6* 67* 69* 68*  0*  0*  3*  0* 97*+32
 4* 5*34*GLAUCOMA        *   1694* 13.1* 75.4*   866* 36.6*   481* 26.4*  2.0* 52* 73* 64*  0*  0*  0*  0*100* 34
 5* 4*96*OTHER INJURY    *   2235* 17.3* 92.7*   233*  9.9*   232* 12.7*  9.6* 79* 73* 73*  4*  0*  0*  0* 96*+96
  *  *  *                *       *      *     *      *      *      *     *     *   *   *   *   *   *   *   *   *
 6* 6* 9*OTHER INF/PARASIT *  265*  2.0* 94.7*    16*   .7*    15*   .8* 16.6* 51* 43* 48*  6*  0*  0*  0* 94*  9
 7* 7*19*OTHER MALIGNANCY  *  218*  1.7* 96.4*    37*  1.6*    33*  1.8*  5.9* 89* 90* 89*  0*  0* 24*  0* 76*+19
 8* 8*83*CONGENITAL DEFECTS*  134*  1.0* 97.4*    47*  2.0*    46*  2.5*  2.9* 72* 78* 78*  0*  0* 13*  0* 87*+83
 9*10*23*DIABETUS MELLITUS *  102*   .8* 98.2*   156*  6.6*   127*  7.0*   .7* 75* 98* 98*  0*  0*  8*  0* 92*+23
10* 9*92*BURN                 109*   .8* 99.0*    11*   .5*    10*   .5*  9.9* 96* 92* 91*  9*  0*  0* 18* 73* 92
  *  *  *                *       *      *     *      *      *      *     *     *   *   *   *   *   *   *   *   *
11*13*86*OTHER UNDIAG SYMP *   14*   .1* 99.1*    28*  1.2*    23*   .3*    .5* 14* 70* 68*  0*  0*  7*  0* 93* 86
12*11*21*OTHER BENIGN TUM  *   55*   .4* 99.5*    30*  1.3*    22*  1.2*  1.8* 71* 86* 81*  0*  0* 23*  0* 77* 21
13*12*46*OTHER CIRC DIS  *     22*   .2* 99.7*     3*   .1*     2*   .1*  7.3* 59* 75* 67*  0*  0*  0*  0*100* 46
14*--*27*MENTAL DERANGE  *   -   *   -  *  -  *  -   *   -  *  -   *  -  *  -  * - * - * - * - * - * - * - * - * 27
15*15*87*SKULL FRACTURE  *      7*   .1* 99.8*     2*   .1*     2*   .1*  3.5* 50* 50* 50*  0*  0*  0*  0*100* 87
  *  *  *                *       *      *     *      *      *      *     *     *   *   *   *   *   *   *   *   *
16*14*22*THYROTOXICOSIS  *     13*   .1* 99.9*     4*   .2*     3*   .2*  3.2*100*100*100*  0*  0* 75*  0* 25* 22
17*18*78*OTHER SKIN DIS  *      2*   .0* 99.9*     4*   .2*     4*   .2*   .5* 33* 80* 80*  0*  0*  0*  0*100* 78
18*16*51*OTHER RESP DIS         4*   .0* 99.9*     1*   .0*     1*   .1*  4.0*100*100*100*  0*  0*  0*  0*100* 51
19*17*94*INTOX CHEMICALS *      4*   .0* 99.9*     1*   .0*     1*   .1*  4.0*100*100*100*  0*  0*  0*  0*100* 94
20*--*39*HYPERTENSION    *   -   *   -  *  -  *  -   *   -  *  -   *  -  *  -  * - * - * - * - * - * - * - * - *
  *  *  *                *       *      *     *      *      *      *     *     *   *   *   *   *   *   *   *   *
21*19*24*OTHER           *      0*   .0* 99.9*     6*   .3*     5*   .3*    .0* - *100*100*  0*  0*  0*  0*100* 24
22*20*75*INFEC SKIN DIS  *      0*   .0* 99.9*     1*   .0*     1*   .1*    .0* - *100*100*  0*  0*  0*  0*100* 75
23*21*79*RHEUMATOID ARTHR *     0*   .0* 99.9*     2*   .1*     1*   .1*    .0* - *100*100*  0*  0*  0*  0*100* 79
24*22*93*INTOX DRUG      *      0*   .0* 99.9*     1*   .0*     1*   .1*    .0* - *100*100*  0*  0*  0*  0*100* 93
25*23*98*PREVENTIVE PROD *      0*   .0* 99.9*     2*   .1*     2*   .1*    .0* - *100*100*  0*  0*100*  0*  0* 98
  *  *  *                *       *      *     *      *      *      *     *     *   *   *   *   *   *   *   *   *
******************************************************************************************************************
TOTAL                    *  12939*100   *100  *  2364*100   *  1822*100  *  5.5* 54* 67* 63*  1*  0*  3*  0* 96*
******************************************************************************************************************
```

FIG 11-1 ILLUSTRATION OF '99' REPORT

across the County, within the unit and within the specialty across the County, are given successively in the first three columns. Naturally there can be a big discrepancy between the latter and its predecessors because of the greater selectivity of the sub-specialty. In the example of an eye clinic shown in Fig 11-1, the top four diagnoses rank similarly across all ophthalmology units but well down the surgical list, while only one of the top twenty surgical diagnoses, and that the rather general one of other infectious parasitic disease, has any occurrence at this clinic.

The ordering of diagnoses in the '99' report is that of the ranking within the sub-specialty or for aggregate specialty reports, within the specialty. Following identification of the diagnoses each line shows

- ward days - number then percentage, the latter being also accumulated
- cases - number then percentage
- patients - number then percentage (i.e. counting only once a patient that presents more than once in the period)
- average length of stay
- percentage of County - for ward days, cases and patients, that this unit provided out of all such within the sub-specialty
- distribution by admission condition - i.e. percentage of cases for each diagnosis that were admitted as emergency from home, emergency other, normal from home, normal other, and not known.

The specialty ranking number is repeated to complete the line. After a final detail line that would hold any unranked diagnoses, the overall picture for the unit is given in a total line.

Besides the internal operational data thus available to each unit, the '99' report thereby provides useful comparative data on both the disease mix and the handling of patients. Hence a unit can, for instance, compare its length-of-stay figures with those of other units while averting false comparisons arising from distinctively different mixes.

The '999' reports - illustrated in Fig 11-2 - carry diagnosis to a deeper level of differentiation. Despite any suggestion to the contrary, the 999 diagnoses of this report are not ten sub-groupings of each of the 99 diagnosis groups of the earlier report, but a varied sub-division of them. Grouped and presented in the order of the 99-level ranking, these finer diagnoses then show the 999-level ranking number, then follow the disease name with similar information on ward days, cases, patients, length of stay and admission condition, but without comparative figures with the wider scene. The report also includes distribution figures on discharge condition - between home, dead, other, and not known. A final column shows non-acute foreigners treated.

Various alternative cross-tabulations and analyses related to these two basic reports are also provided, e.g. analyzing discharges by sex and age band, at the 99-level.

Special Analyses

The exceptional aggregation of both medical data and extensive sociological/census data on a complete regional population provides opportunity for far-ranging studies on morbidity and health-care utilization. However, the recency of wide implementation of the key inpatient sub-system and the moratorium on extending other sub-systems limits the extent to which such potential can yet be realized.

STOCKHOLM COUNTY COUNCIL
HEALTH- AND MEDICAL-CARE
CENTRAL OFFICE
OPERATIONS DEPT

INPATIENT DISCHARGES DURING 1971 — 999-LIST — PAGE 1

SPECIALTY: INTERNAL MEDICINE — MEDICINE DEPT
SUBSPECIALTY: GENERAL MEDICINE — DANDERYD HOSPITAL

DIAG CODE 99	999	NAME	STAY DAYS NUMBER	STAY DAYS %	CASES	PAT-IENTS	MEAN STAY DAYS	ADMISSION CONDN % ACUTE HOM	ACUTE OTH	NON-ACU HOM	NON-ACU OTH	NOT KNW	DISCHARGE CONDN % HOM	D'D	OTH	NOT KNW	% NON ACUT FRGN
2		ENTERIC DIARRHOEA	132	100	20	19	6.6	55	0	40	5	0	80	0	20	0	-
	009	INFEC GAST ENT	132	100	20	19	6.6	55	0	40	5	0	80	0	20	0	
3		TB IN RESP ORGAN	49	100	4	4	12.2	100	0	0	0	0	75	0	25	0	-
	011	TB PULM	15	31	3	3	5.0	100	0	0	0	0	67	0	33	0	-
	012	TB RESP OTHER	34	69	1	1	34.0	100	0	0	0	0	100	0	0	0	-
4		OTHER TB SEQUELAE	64	100	4	2	16.0	100	0	0	0	0	50	0	50	0	-
	016	TB URO-GENITAL SEQ	41	64	3	1	13.7	100	0	0	0	0	67	0	33	0	-
	019	TB OTHER SEQUELAE	23	36	1	1	23.0	100	0	0	0	0	0	0	100	0	-
5		STREPTOCCAL THROAT	23	100	1	1	23.0	0	0	100	0	0	100	0	0	0	-
	034	STREP THROAT	23	100	1	1	23.0	0	0	100	0	0	100	0	0	0	-
6		INFEC HEPATITIS	6	100	2	1	3.0	100	0	0	0	0	100	0	0	0	-
	070	HEPATITIS	6	100	2	1	3.0	100	0	0	0	0	100	0	0	0	-
9		OTHER INF OR PARASIT	275	100	33	26	8.3	73	3	24	0	0	82	6	12	0	-
	035	ERYSIPELAS	105	38	12	9	8.7	92	8	0	0	0	92	0	8	0	-
	036	MENINGEOCOCC	0	0	1	1	.0	100	0	0	0	0	0	100	0	0	-
	044	POLIO AFTER-EFFECT	39	14	1	1	39.0	100	0	0	0	0	0	0	100	0	-
	045	MENING ENTEROVIR	3	1	3	2	1.0	100	0	0	0	0	67	0	33	0	-
	053	SHINGLES	24	9	2	1	12.0	100	0	0	0	0	50	0	50	0	-
	079	OTHER VIRUS DIS	8	3	4	4	2.0	75	0	25	0	0	100	0	0	0	-
	131	TRICHOM URO-GEN	2	1	1	1	2.0	100	0	0	0	0	100	0	0	0	-
	135	SARCOIDOSIS	94	34	9	7	10.4	22	0	78	0	0	89	11	0	0	-

FIG 11-2 ILLUSTRATION OF '999' REPORT

Currently two distinct types of special analyses are performed. One pertains to the patients of one particular doctor or clinic and is done at the request of the doctor concerned. The other is more general, initiated by the County authorities. Both apply to the H.R., but can extend into the archival Patient History files.

A doctor-requested analysis is essentially a selective search. It is requisitioned and specified by a form that, upon completion, is vetted by the Information Systems Bureau before submission to the computer. The form lists 18 variables pertaining to inpatient recordss and 12 pertaining to x-ray record that can be cited as selection parameters and/or for output use. These cover birthdate, age and sex of patient, hospital department and clinic of service, date of service, and the various codes for procedures and findings. An 'x' in the appropriate square indicates use in selection: a circle around the square indicates use in output. The actual values for selection parameters are specified in the lower part of the form, and can be single values, or whole or broken ranges, with equalities or inequalities. The search can be specified as being of a given time point, and to be inclusive or exclusive of patients removed from the H.R. It can also be restricted to particular areas for home address. The report can be either a statistical tabulation or a listing of cases, and the order within such a list is specifiable.

The first major general study was performed during 1975, relative to 1973, and was of health-care utilization. Perhaps the first such comprehensive regional study ever conducted, it showed large variations in the level of utilization between the residents of the score of municipalities that make up the County, and even between the numerous parishes of Stockholm municipality. The availability of the detailed address/locational data in the CFU records allowed this geographical analysis, while availability of corresponding demographic data for each area allowed the utilization data to be put into an age/sex context. Differing age profiles in different areas were insufficient to account for the different levels of utilization; nor were different availabilities of service seen as crucial. Both environmental and occupational factors were seen as influential, but neither could be methodically accommodated in this pioneer study.

CHAPTER 12

SECURITY

Beyond the security provided by the closely controlled data centre and the oversight of most terminals, the overall security is dependent on the use of enciphered identity numbers for each approved user of the System.

Each approved user is registered within the System with an internal security code that includes the following fields, of sizes shown: 3 bits, overall category (i.e., computer staff, health care staff, county housing authority staff, health insurance organization staff); 4 bits, institution (in particular, hospital or hospital group); 6 bits, department (or clinic) within institution; 7 bits, individual's number within department; 1 bit, whether individual is restricted to terminals within cited department; 2 bits, security level of user, and 1 bit, whether individual is restricted to information generated by this cited department.

These fields are assembled in one 30-bit computer word, the balance of which is used for associated purposes. The individual's number mentioned is not one used generally, but one assigned purely for this purpose. It differentiates individuals having otherwise identical characteristics, and also allows a change of identification for any individual whose external code has become known to another person.

Along with the appropriate values for these fields, the registration of any user includes entry of personal name, address and date. Provisions for amendment and deletion are also included.

Upon entry or amendment and, periodically as certain common parameters are altered, the computer applies an enciphering algorithm to the aggregate internal security code, producing an external security code. This algorithm initially converts the internal security code to another binary number, its 30-bit word being then interpreted as six 5-bit characters. This appears to the user as an alphanumeric word using a 32-character set of graphics that excludes the more ambivalent graphics.

In practice, the structure of the internal security code and of the algorithm are such that the hospital staff member has only a 5-character external security code.

The computed external security code is printed blind within a sealed envelope, at Datacentral, but the envelope is issued to the user by the security control clerk of the pertinent institution.

Access to the real-time system is then obtained by the user keying the external security code. Communication of this brief message causes the computer to apply the reverse algorithm, then check whether the derived internal security code is in its list of approved codes. Currently the approved users number less than 2 000 so the 5-character code alone provides only a 1-in-16 000 chance of any erroneous or random entry coinciding with an approved code.

An initial failure to hit a valid code results in an appropriate response from the computer, but opportunity to try again. However, repeated failure - currently set at more than four - results in closure of the terminal and the alerting of operational staff. The terminal involved remains closed until an appropriate command is issued by such staff.

Entry of an acceptable security code results in a response at the terminal that shows the last date and time that this code was entered. The System thus provides the means for each user to maintain surveillance over the use of his code, and to detect illicit intrusions.

At this point the user can proceed to enter the code and other details of the first intended transaction, be it an inquiry or an advice. However, the security control is far from finished; as can be presumed from the enunciated components of the internal security code, various controls are applied to the procedures and information that can be accessed.

The computer has knowledge of the location of each terminal, including the department in which it is situated. If a user's security code specifies a restriction to terminals within the department, then an appropriate check is made and failure results in closure of the dialog.

The next stage of control rests with the routines called as a consequence of the transaction code entered. Each application routine has the latitude to apply whatever controls are deemed appropriate for it. Likewise control is applied selectively to the acquisition and use of information from the various files. This control is selective by file, by field, and even according to values of fields. Control over procedures and information is never dependent on the individual's number within the security code, but only on the generic components.

While the H.R. is accessible to virtually all users, at least to some extent, the majority of files pertain to either an individual hospital or an equivalent group. Access to them is therefore restricted to users having the corresponding institution code. In contrast, access to the procedural routines is controlled overall by the user's overall category.

More detailed control over both procedure and information is based on user security level. The four discrete levels established, are: level 1: users needing access only to basic identification and sociological data, in H.R. and for patient files, e.g., admission clerks, reception/information staff; level 2: users needing access to hospital attendance data and critical medical information, e.g., nursing personnel, medical and ward secretaries; level 3: users needing diagnoses and other medical data, e.g., medical and emergency department staff, and level 4: not currently defined.

These levels are obviously defined within the context of hospital category users. The non-hospital users are essentially level 1 at present, and labelled as such; one or more distinctive series of level definitions could be developed for them in due course, to operate only within the context of their categories.

Table 12-1 summarizes the availability of information to users of the different levels, respectively, for the H.R. and for the pertinent patient file.

It must be noted in Table 12-1 that the availability of certain

LEVEL	H.R.	P.R.
3	INPATIENT AND X-RAY INFORMATION, INCLUSIVE OF DIAGNOSES AND VERBAL NOTES	
2	INPATIENT AND X-RAY INFORMATION EXCLUDING DIAGNOSES AND SIMILAR MEDICAL DATA	DETAILED MEDICAL INFORMATION FROM USER'S OWN DEPARTMENT
1	BASIC SOCIOLOGICAL DATA	ATTENDANCE INFORMATION, PLUS DIAGNOSES FROM USER'S DEPARTMENT

TABLE 12-1 AVAILABILITY OF INFORMATION ON H.R. AND P.R. TO USERS WITH DIFFERENT SECURITY LEVELS.

information from the patient files is restricted to users from the originating department. Thus, for instance, a member of the medical department is precluded from accessing medical details originating in the surgical department. Admitting clerks are effectively precluded from accessing any such data. However, since clinical laboratory reports are effectively tagged as belonging to the requisitioning department, so as to be accessible to members of that department, the laboratory staff themselves are accorded all-department status. This is achieved by setting the pertinent constituent of the security code to show them, abnormally, as not restricted to information generated in their own department. This overrides any marking for departmental dependence shown as required within a file.

The accessibilities described above and summarized in the table need to be further qualified in regard to certain attendances and diagnoses deemed 'sensitive'. Attendance at a veneral diseases or psychiatric clinic, and the diagnosis of abortion or attempted suicide are examples of 'sensitive' information. Generally, such information is unavailable via the real-time terminals; it is obtainable through the further scrutiny applicable to submissions to the batch processes.

This control of access to sensitive entries is clearly less systematic than the preceding controls, and requires exhaustive reference to a table of prohibitions. While necessarily expensive, it could be extended indefinitely to meet other selective prohibitions.

It may be observed that no control is made on the basis of individual patient or individual user. There is, for instance, no control over the patient records accessed within a department by a particular doctor. Any attempt by a user to access information that is precluded only by departmental and/or level incompatibilities results in a response stating the inaccessibility.

To minimize the risk of illicit use of valid external security codes, all codes are collectively annulled periodically and replaced by new codes calculated with changed parameters in the algorithm. The change of code by each user must be made at the common gazetted time, to accord with the implementation of the corresponding change in the deciphering algorithm.

Where knowledge or even suspicion warrants it, any user can at any time seek annulment of the currently assigned external code and its replacement by another. The alteration is achieved by replacement of the individual number in the registered internal code. Though representing one distinct fragment of the total internal code, the enciphering algorithm is designed to spread its effect over the whole external code. This means not only that the one user receives an overall new code in his special situation, but also that there is no 'family likeness' of codes within a department.

Legal Constraints and Obligations

Prompted largely by the growing concern, felt internationally, regarding the threat of computers to privacy and confidentiality, the Swedish parliament ('Riksdag') passed, in 1973, a bill that regulates the use of computers with personal information. Though a fairly common reaction to a very common concern, Sweden had a rather distinctive need for such legislation because of the long-standing tradition of freedom of information. Based on an initial promulgation of 1766, the Freedom-of-the-Press Act provides, in what is called the 'publicity-principle', a general right of the public to see and even have copies of documents held by the government. Exception can be made explicitly, and is made, under a Secrecy Act, of documents relating to such things as personal medical, social or financial data, combatting crime, and various aspects of military and foreign affairs. However, computers offered scope to assemble the myriads of information that are so available in a manner potentially prejudicial to privacy.

The new act, referred to as the Swedish Data Act, is aimed at preventing unacceptable intrusions into privacy without impairing the traditional freedom of information. To achieve this, the Act established a Data Inspection Board empowered to supervise and control the creation, maintenance and use of files of personal information. The Act provides that such personal files can exist only with the approval of the Board, and under conditions enunciated by the Board. 'Personal file' is defined to include any index, list or other notes, kept with the aid of computer processing, that contains any particular concerning individual people. It follows that such things as car registrations and registers of real property are personal files if they contain any data about the owner.

In considering any personal file for approval, the Board is concerned with its proposed contents and uses, the apparent attitudes and responsibility of the party proposing to keep the file, and the perceived attitude of the people that would be included therein. The Act does not require the agreement, or even perceived agreement or non-objection of the latter. The Act does not even require that there be no intrusion, but merely that there be no improper or unnecessary intrusion into personal privacy. But it does require adequate reason for the file - a facet particularly restrictive to parties other than public authorities charged by law with the maintenance of such files.

Illnesses and other health matters, political beliefs of affiliations, and religious convictions are matters of particular concern. Beyond the keeping of mere membership lists by political or religious organizations and the keeping of medical records by pertinent authorities, very special grounds are required for the inclusion of such data in files.

The Act requires the checking of any item of personal data suspected to be in error, and the removal of any item that is apparently erroneous. If the erroneous item has been provided to others, appropriate corrective action must be taken, unless special exemption is made by the Board. Similar responsibilities are placed on the holding party concerning omissions if these can be deleterious to privacy or rights of the person concerned. The Act explicitly forbids the supply of any information to a third party if there is reason to suspect that it will be used illegally. All staff involved with the data must observe professional secrecy regarding the data and the knowledge it provides.

As a means of ensuring both the continued attendance to rules and regulations for approved files and the detection of illegal personal files, the Board has the power to inspect any data processing installation in Sweden, though it must confine its activities to the field of personal data and privacy. The person responsible for any approved personal file must provide, and ensure that any third party such as a computer service bureau provide any documentation or other evidence required by the Board.

The Act also provides the right of any individual included in the file to know the data recorded as pertaining to him. The general provision is that such data be provided at least once per year, upon request, in reasonable hard copy form and free of inhibitory charge - indeed gratuitously if possible.

The new act contains various penal clauses, with fines and/or gaol sentences for general infringements. It also creates, additional to offences included in the criminal code, a new category of crime 'data trespass'. This covers unlawful altering or erasing of personal data, and carries a sentence of up to 2 years imprisonment and/or a fine. Civil liability to the persons in the register is also established in the Act, with non-pecuniary consequences being assessable.

Should a responsible party wish or be obliged to discontinue maintenance of a personal file, the disposal of the data is to be at the direction of the Board.

The Stockholm County Medical System, in the continuation of the well-established traditions for confidentiality of medical records, had a substantial security component included in it from the outset. However, the new Data Act necessitated some adjustments, as well as the formalities for approval.

In conformity with the Act, any patient can receive a copy of his record upon request (once yearly). The procedure provides for the non-medical information to be sent directly to the patient, by ordinary mail, from Datacentral. The medical information, however, is forwarded to last the updating department for verification prior to dispatch via 'special delivery' mail. The overall system operates on the principle that each medical department must have reasonable confidence in the existing medical data before adding to it, so ostensibly only the last entry needs scrutiny at any point. However, any department can, at any time, seek verification of any entry by the originating department. No charge is made for providing the information to the patient.

CHAPTER 13

IMPLEMENTING THE SYSTEM

Initial implementation

Following trial use of the earliest sub-systems from 1969 on, the first official implementation occurred, with the waiting list and inpatient sub-systems, in the Danderyd hospital in June 1971. Expansion beyond this acute general hospital, which had been the scene of the trials and the source of the System, followed in late 1971. The inpatient sub-system was implemented during October in the 3,000-bed psychiatric hospital Beckomberga and the waiting list sub-system in the largest general hospital of Stockholm City - Soder hospital. This expansion thus took both initial sub-systems beyond their pilot home, and also brought example of each being used without the other, albeit for practical reasons - there being no waiting list for psychiatric patients and considerable difficulties facing the introduction of the inpatient sub-system at Soder which, unlike Danderyd, was a fully established rather than expanding hospital.

The wholly new Huddinge hospital was due to open, equipped with the computerized information system, in 1972, and expansion of the System to several other hospitals was also planned for late that year. Based on the experience gained with the less-formally planned early implementations, careful plans were laid for these extensions.

Strategy for implementation

Because of the large numbers of patients waiting for admission to each general hospital, it was decided to make the waiting list sub-system the initial step for each hospital. Ten terminals were installed over eight hospitals for this purpose, continuing until the back-log of listings was cleared in 1973. Only four were necessary for the on-going work after conversion.

The inpatient sub-system was seen as the next logical step. Because of its pervasive influence, this sub-system requires extensive preparation prior to implementation in any hospital. Preparation must be started 12 months before the proposed conversion date, with meetings between central and local staffs, both managerial and operational. Since each hospital presents its own distinctive problems to add to the common problems of understanding and detailed technical implementation, two study groups are formed at this initial stage - one for technical matters of installation and one for internal systems aspects for the hospital. Each group must survey its respective situation and have its plans, including proposed adaptations to meet local variations, ready for approval 6 months prior to the scheduled conversion date. For the technical group the plans must cover location of terminals and associated communications units, plus routing of lines. For the implementation group routine matters include the assignment of codes, the cut-over plans and the education of staff.

Approval of these plans must be given by the hospital administration and the central staff of the Health Department, i.e. the Information Systems Bureau; where program alterations are necessary, it must also be obtained from Datacentral, who must in any case concur with the operational impact. The Bureau, responsible in the beginning for system specifications, is responsible for general acceptance testing and then for implementation. The Director of the Bureau - a physician with over 10 years of expérience in the County hospitals, has two assistants concerned with oversighting this implementation work, plus five instructors that teach terminal users. The two assistants cover the technical installation and the system implementation fields respectively, and lead the respective study groups.

Education of the hospital staff begins in general at this mid-year point, through the hospital's staff newspaper. Three months later this process is repeated with expanded information, while briefing sessions are also held with the various labor organizations. Where the hospital has its own internal T.V. channel, this medium is used too, usually about one month prior to cut-over.

This timetable of informing hospital staff is carefully drawn to provide adequate forewarning without a premature overloading with detail. Regarding the former facet, it should be noted that the labor organizations involved have been advised, at their central office for the Department, far in advance of these developments, and accord reached on the industrial questions involved. Training of staff in terminal usage, on the other hand, begins with only three weeks left to cutover, in accordance with the above principle but also so as to minimize wastage and to make best use of the terminals. Since, as discussed below, the training schedule requires just three weeks, this arrangement means that the newly trained staff put their training to immediate use, maximizing the effectiveness of the training. Motivation of the trainees is also optimal at this juncture.

Implementation timetable to 1975

Table 13-1 shows the timetable for implementation through 1976 and how, after Huddinge in March 72 (and excluding its subsequent expansions), the inpatient sub-system was not introduced to any further hospital until December 74. In the meantime, coverage of the waiting list had been considerably extended. The extension of the chemical laboratory sub-system to Beckomberga, which remains the only such implementation other than Huddinge, is the only exception in a long sequence of waiting list implementations. Except for the Karolinska, which was not integrated into the County operations until 1975, the year 1974 saw completion of conversion of the vast majority of the waiting list and 1975 was devoted to implementation of the inpatient sub-system.

After Huddinge, neither the booking nor the outpatient sub-system has been implemented, except for a limited case at the Karolinska, which was the birthplace of the booking sub-system. This paucity reflects opinion on the relative merits and respective difficulties of each sub-system.

A summary of the current implementation situation, with indications of the sizes of the separate hospitals, is shown in Table 13-2.

The arrangement for cut-over

The cut-over of any hospital to the inpatient sub-system must be done at one time for the whole hospital (or at least very major parts thereof), and with a very clear demarcation between 'before' and 'after'. All such cutovers are made as Sunday changes to Monday. Though the influx of

DATE	INSTITUTION	SUB-SYSTEM
JUN 71	DANDERYD	W,I
OCT 71	BECKOMBERGA	I
NOV 71	SODER	W
DEC 71	DUNDERYD	B
MAR 72	HUDDINGE*	W,I,B(RADIOL & INT. MED), O,C
JUN 72	ST. ERIK'S	W
SEP 72	SABBATSBERG	W
OCT 72	BECKOMBERGA	C
OCT 72	NACKA	W
OCT 72	ERSTA	W
NOV 72	ST. GORAN'S	W (ADULTS)
FEB 73	ST. GORAN'S	W (CHILDREN)
FEB 73	LOWENSTROMSKA	W
DEC 74	SODERTALJE	W
DEC 74	SODER	I
MAR 75	SODERTALJE	I
AUG 75	KAROLINSKA	W
SEP 75	KAROLINSKA	I
OCT 75	KAROLINSKA	B (PULM. & T.B. FELLO REP)
OCT 75	ST. ERIK'S	I
NOV 75	SABBATSBERG	I
MAR 76	ROSLAGSTULL	I
APR 76	ST. GORAN'S	I

TABLE 13-1 THE PROGRESS OF IMPLEMENTATION TO MID '76.

SEE TABLE 13-2 FOR DATA ON HOSPITAL SIZES.

*HUDDINGE HAD ONLY 100 BEDS WHEN OPENED IN MAR 72. EXPANSION TO 400 BEDS OCCURRED IN OCT 72 AND TO 800 IN 1974; CONCOMITANT EXPANSION OF COMPUTER TERMINAL NETWORK AND FILE COVERAGE OCCURRED ON EACH OCCASION.

NEITHER THE PSYCHIATRIC HOSPITAL AT BECKOMBERGA NOR THE INFECTIOUS DISEASES ONE AT ROSLAGSTULL HAS WAITING PATIENTS.

elective patients during Sunday typically means that the hospital population is not minimal at that instant, the choice minimizes the problem of having pertinent records up-to-date. Every effort is made to have the record of each current inpatient brought up-to-date during the Friday and Saturday, particularly as regards continuing patients. The patient lists distributed on Sunday morning, reflecting the status to the preceding midnight, are carefully scrutinized, and corrected, during that afternoon. Thus, together with the diligently recorded new day's admission, Monday can open with the current patient population correctly recorded in the computer system. Simultaneously responsibility switches, the visiting implementation team, which had handled the conversion, passing responsibility for terminal operation to the normal hospital staff. However, the implementation team must remain on-hand until assured that the local staff are able to operate without the outside supervision and help. It is often a month before the last of this outside team leaves the hospital.

Education of users

The implementation of any new procedures or systems demands some familiarization of involved personnel if success is to be achieved. For a real-time computer system those demands are clearly much more intensive, particularly where, as in Stockholm the computer processes are vital to the immediate and on-going operation of the facilities.

	TYPE	BEDS	PATIENTS WAITING	ANNUAL ADMISSIONS	FIRST DATE	SUBSYSTEMS
DANDERYD	G	1 047	1 879	28 000	1971	I, B
BECKOMBERGA	A	1 519		3 000	1971	I, L
HUDDINGE	G	795	2 521	21 000	1972	I, O, L, B
SODER	G	1 329	3 723	35 000	1972	I
KAROLINSKA	G	1 176	1 000	39 000	1975	I
ST ERIK	G	528	1 176	15 000	1972	I
SABBATSBERG	G	658	2 163	16 000	1972	I
ST GORAN	G	766	2 134	17 000	1973	I (1976)
LOWEN	G	447	257	9 000	1973	I (1976)
NACKA	G	348	348	11 000	1973	I
SODERTALJE	G	437	279	11 000	1973	I
SERAFIMER	G	535	302	9 000	1974	I (1967)

TABLE 13-2 CURRENT IMPLEMENTATION STATUS

SHOWS NUMBERS OF BEDS, ADMISSIONS AND WAITING PATIENTS.
THE "FIRST DATE" GENERALLY INDICATES INCORPORATION WITH THE WAITING LIST.

A = ACUTE PSYCHIATRIC HOSPITAL
G = GENERAL HOSPITAL (USUALLY INCLUDES SOME LONG-TERM BEDS)
I = INPATIENT ROUTINE
O = OUTPATIENT ROUTINE
L = LABORATORY ROUTINE
B = BOOKING ROUTINE

Though thousands of medical, nursing, administrative and other staff are affected by the new developments, from first steps with input data to using reports, the direct use of the terminals has, by an early decision, been much more restricted. While an explicit terminal operator classification has not been created, the security needs and measures alone point to a distinct corps of approved users. These comprise nurses plus clerical and secretarial staff mainly - particularly ward and medical secretaries - with laboratory technicians making up most of the balance. Very few medical staff have been direct users of the terminals. Education hence needs to be deep and thorough for only a modicum of staff, with widespread education only in the appreciation sense.

The start of the widespread education occurs through the in-house news media already mentioned. A 1-hour introductory talk (shown in Fig 13-1 as the first step in more detailed training, and embedded in Module 1 of Fig 13-2 regarding the current training scheme) is given for all staff affected, and specific training sessions, plus pertinent written instructions, provided for staff affected by changes in forms, and equivalent procedures. A special talk for physicians is given by the Director of the Information Systems Bureau; however, as their use of the System is almost always through such an intermediary as a receptionist, nurse or secretary, it is the latter people rather than physicians that have been taught to use the System. However, there is a growing interest, plus an intention to use the terminals themselves, among younger physicians and increasing attention is being given to teaching physicians the detailed use of the terminals and the facilities offered. The research analyses available only through the batch route are, of course, of distinct interest to the medical staffs.

The specific training of staff in the use of the terminals, involving knowledge of the hardware, the programmed procedures for its general use, the security system, and the explicit details of the pertinent dialogs, has been mentioned as taking three weeks. The training methods and objectives have been varied over the years, and that is the current scheme.

<u>Original training scheme</u>

When the System was implemented initially at Danderyd, the hospital staff were told how to operate the terminals, and how to use the System, by the various programmers concerned. The students were taught individually, each having a terminal. This arrangement was neither efficient nor very effective. The typical programmer had neither a common language with his student nor a compatible understanding and outlook. Nor had he necessarily any aptitude for teaching. The result was an expensive failure that had the additional disadvantage of fostering an antagonism to the System within the hospital staff.

<u>Creation of training unit</u>

Such bad experince led quickly to the establishment of a small training unit, staffed with people able to acquire the knowledge from the programmers and able to pass this on reasonably easily to the numerous nurses, secretaries and others that must operate the System. To ensure compatibility between the training unit staff (instructors) and the students, the staff for this new unit were chosen from the nurses, doctor's secretaries and ward secretaries who showed aptitude for this new field. The five staff selected were given an extensive education in general aspects of e.d.p. as well as the particulars for the County, covering six months. They were then deployed not only to training of intended terminal users, but as the implementation field force that works with their graduates to bring each new implementation to successful running. (The group still numbers five, though the means for refilling vacancies are naturally somewhat changed.)

This new unit was used for the first time with the introduction of the System to Huddinge for which, in conjunction with educational specialists, it developed a formal training programme and materials. This programme consisted of three phases.

The first phase, lasting only one hour, was the general introduction for all staff in the hospital.

The second phase - a training programme for those who have to work either with computer printouts or terminals - introduced the trainees to the terminals, the H.R. and its associated dialogs, the P.R., and cursorily to each sub-system. At its end the trainees were conversant with the overall and general aspects, including practical use of a terminal. Phase II took about nine hours of assigned time.

Phase II took the trainees more deeply into their respective areas of concern, taking four to eight hours depending on the sub-system.

The layout and content of this education plan is shown in Fig 13-1. The teaching was assisted by audiovisual aids and special procedures to allow exercise use of the terminals, and augmented by instruction books

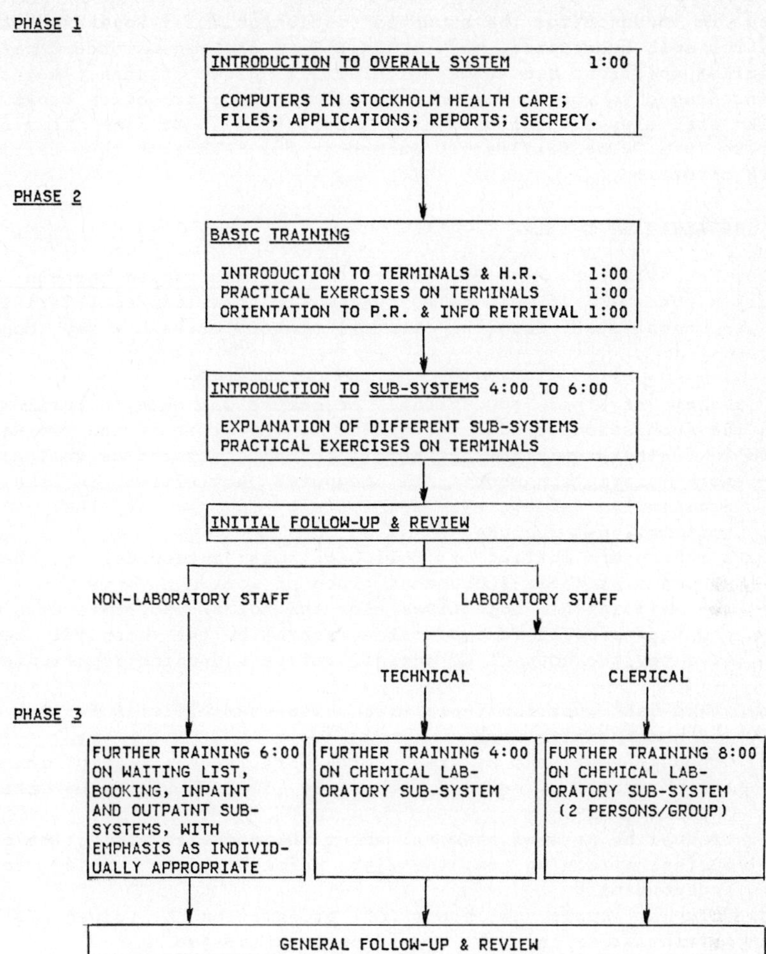

FIG 13-1 TRAINING PROGRAMME - 1972 EDITION

(PUNCTUATED NUMBERS SHOW HRS:MINS ASSIGNED)

prepared in advance for the students' individual use. Separate books were written for each sub-system, each organized to the same standard pattern so that similar questions are answered in similar parts of each. The students were encouraged to work independently with these instruction books, copies of which are always available, as appropriate, at the terminals in productive use. The familiarity gained in the classroom thus carries into the work situation.

Review and revision - 1973

From Feb 1972 thru May 1973 about 800 students passed through courses of this nature, 58% of them being nurses, 29% clerical/secretarial staff, and 13% technical staff from the chemical laboratories, x-ray department and such.

A review of this educational structure was made in April/May 1973 through the submission of a questionnaire to the staff it had trained. This resulted in further revision, the programme being altered as follows,

- more information about all computer activities in the field, especially about all sub-systems in use at the particular hospital, was included
- a scheme of instructor follow-up was introduced to help the students at their subsequent place of work
- the attainment objectives for the formal programme were defined and made subject to explicit agreement by the hospital concerned (i.e. by the council of administrative and union representatives).

For this last question there were three possibilities for the overall objective of the formal course

a) Graduating persons be ready to work independently immediately after training, except for only the odd follow-up visit by an instructor
b) Graduating persons know all about the computer activities but need further training on the job before being able to work independently
c) Only a couple of hours of orientation be given, with all particular training to be effected on-the-job.

Though the first of these possibilities entails the largest explicit cost for training, the other two were estimated to have higher real costs through the inefficiency of instruction plus the protracted period of marginal utility of each on-the-job trainee. Any use of the System by a part-trained person must carry a relative high risk of error, while the instruction gained by such a trainee is itself more likely to be erroneous than instruction from a select person expressly obliged to be correct in every detail. Hence, alternative (a), which is really the only viable one for new implementations, was adjudged to be preferable generally, and so was adopted. While each newly graduating person must be given time in the productive setting to achieve full productivity, this choice meant that the numbers to be trained could be related closely to the estimated workload.

The investigation also brought the following changes:-

- supplementing of direct instruction with more self-directed study, appropriate material being prepared and provided; this allowed 10 students to be trained by one instructor, with increased individual follow-up to obviate problems absorbing the saved

effort, and allowed pairs of students to share a terminal in most courses
- an increase in the practical examples to be completed by each student, plus the introduction of frequent tests on the student's progress in practical competence
- a final examination that the student has to pass in order to complete successfully the course.

About 90% of the pupils pass the final examination at the first attempt, and about half the balance succeed at a subsequent attempt. The external security code, essential for use of a terminal, is assigned only after the passing of this examination. Students that fail this hurdle cannot be employed as intended; because they have usually been given an appointment to the pertinent job classification before entry upon the course, they must therefore be found equivalent employment in a situation not requiring System-user status. While such openings will likely become less with time, this has presented no difficulty to date.

Initially after introduction of the final examination this problem of job placement was avoided by allowing everyone to proceed along the intended path irrespective of examination result, but experience soon pointed to such a practice being a mistake.

The content of the course remained virtually unchanged by these revisions, but the layout was altered to that depicted in Fig 13-2.

Over 400 students have attended this style of course over the last three years, covering both additional hospitals and replacement staff. Of these about 60% were nurses, 25% clerical/secretarial and 15% laboratory staff - the changed composition being due in part to the fact that the x-ray and laboratory applications have not been extended beyond the early examples.

<u>On-going education and assistance to users</u>

The proliferation of terminals and the extension of the System to many hospitals has brought a district organization to act as a bridge between the central staff and the hundreds of hospital employees that are now users of the System.

Four of the five County districts have now an E.D.P. Assistant, in some cases with one or two additional staff. These people help hospital staff deal with emergent problems, help them avoid potential problems, acquaint them with changes and developments in the System, and, where necessary, act as relief staff.

The district staff meet every other week with the central staff, gaining knowledge of forthcoming changes and at the same time feeding back the views and ideas of the users.

Changes in the System are advised in written form one to two weeks in advance of effect, with memoranda and/or insertions for the user manual issued as appropriate. Responsibility for user documentation rests with the system implementation assistant at the Bureau.

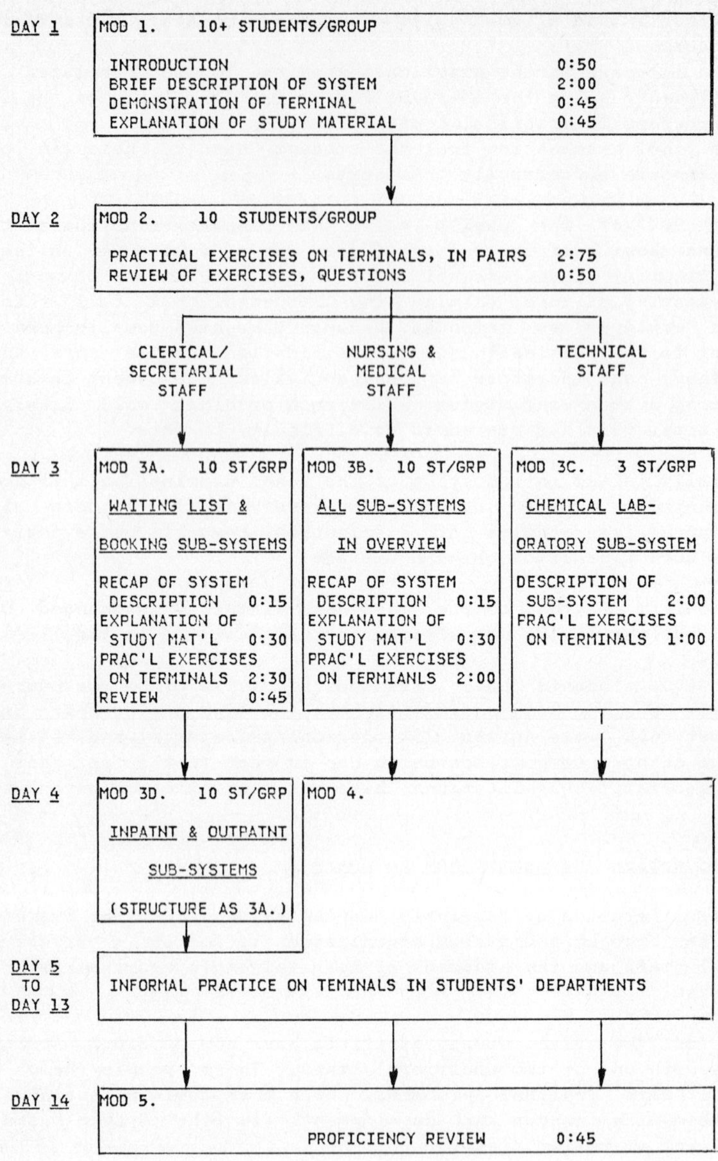
DAY 1
MOD 1. 10+ STUDENTS/GROUP
INTRODUCTION 0:50
BRIEF DESCRIPTION OF SYSTEM 2:00
DEMONSTRATION OF TERMINAL 0:45
EXPLANATION OF STUDY MATERIAL 0:45
DAY 2
MOD 2. 10 STUDENTS/GROUP
PRACTICAL EXERCISES ON TERMINALS, IN PAIRS 2:75
REVIEW OF EXERCISES, QUESTIONS 0:50
CLERICAL/ SECRETARIAL STAFF
NURSING & MEDICAL STAFF
TECHNICAL STAFF
DAY 3
MOD 3A. 10 ST/GRP
WAITING LIST & BOOKING SUB-SYSTEMS
RECAP OF SYSTEM DESCRIPTION 0:15
EXPLANATION OF STUDY MAT'L 0:30
PRAC'L EXERCISES ON TERMINALS 2:30
REVIEW 0:45
MOD 3B. 10 ST/GRP
ALL SUB-SYSTEMS IN OVERVIEW
RECAP OF SYSTEM DESCRIPTION 0:15
EXPLANATION OF STUDY MAT'L 0:30
PRAC'L EXERCISES ON TERMIANLS 2:00
MOD 3C. 3 ST/GRP
CHEMICAL LAB-ORATORY SUB-SYSTEM
DESCRIPTION OF SUB-SYSTEM 2:00
FRAC'L EXERCISES ON TERMINALS 1:00
DAY 4
MOD 3D. 10 ST/GRP
INPATNT & OUTPATNT SUB-SYSTEMS
(STRUCTURE AS 3A.)
MOD 4.
DAY 5 TO DAY 13
INFORMAL PRACTICE ON TEMINALS IN STUDENTS' DEPARTMENTS
DAY 14
MOD 5.
PROFICIENCY REVIEW 0:45

FIG 13-2 TRAINING PROGRAMME - 1973 EDITION

(PUNCTUATED NUMBERS SHOWS HRS:MINS ASSIGNED)

CHAPTER 14

EVALUATIONS AND PLANS

The primary objective of a regional medical information system based on a central population register has undoubtedly been achieved for the Stockholm County. However, while the inpatient sub-system is about to join the waiting list sub-system in having total geographical coverage, the remaining three sub-systems are effectively subject to a moratorium pending development of significantly improved versions. Even with the inpatient sub-system, the functional coverage would be considerable short of what many would require in a reasonably comprehensive system.

Through the consolidated waiting list and the analysis of utilization, the System can already assist materially the planners of health care services - an important objective. For hospital staffs the System provides direct advantages in being a fast, reliable means of processing that helps reduce the clutter and confusion that tends to occur in a busy hospital. But what is this all worth, and what is the cost?

Costs and Benefits of Current System

Unfortunately, despite being in operation for several years, no thorough analysis of costs and benefits has yet been carried out on the System. For one hospital (Soder), a comparison of the real-time inpatient procedures with preceding batch computer processing has been made - with favorable conclusions regarding the newer. But this was both too restricted in its field of study and light in its depth of analysis. The facts that the pilot site was a massive rebuilding project and that the major scene of implementation is a new hospital that has known no other processes make comparative analysis difficult. Just now, in 1976, a major cost/benefit study is being mounted by the County in conjuction with SPRI - the national agency for rationalization in the field of health care.

The total expenditure by Stockholm County on medical E.D.P. over the nine years since the System was initiated has been assessed at over 60 million Swedish crowns, inclusive of development, operations and capital expenditures. Table 14-1 gives the annual figures over these years of both all E.D.P. and the estimated medical share. By 1975 the medical share was virtually half of a 26 million crown total, setting it at about $3 million, representing $2 per capita. (Inflation and fluctuating exchange rates render inappropriate any formal conversion of the Swedish figures. For informal conversion, the Swedish crown can be equated with the French franc, the Swiss franc and German mark equal 2 crowns, the U.S. and Canadian dollars 4 crowns and the English pound 8 crowns.)

It seems very doubtful that such expenditures are covered by tangible savings, and indeed doubtful that the savings would cover even the operational costs, which account for about 85% of current expenditures but a much lower proportion of those past. However, the System was not developed for economic reasons but for improved service to planners, managers, hospital staff and patients. In this regard the System has undoubtedly brought significant benefit. The arbiter of whether the price is worth the gain, currently and in the future, is the Stockholm County

	TOTAL	MEDICAL
1967	1 777	250
1968	4 511	2 000
1969	6 518	3 700
1970	7 497	4 500
1971	12 377	6 200
1972	16 700	9 000
1973	18 724	10 224
1974	24 696	13 527
1975	26 522	13 126

TABLE 14-1 PAST EXPENDITURES ON E.D.P. BY STOCKHOLM COUNTY (EXPRESSED IN THOUSANDS OF CROWNS)

NOTE: MEDICAL SHARES PRIOR TO 1973 ARE BY RETROSPECTIVE ESTIMATE.

Council, and this body has consistently supported both the continuation of the System and its progressive development and extension.

Besides annual budgetting, the Council, as is common in Sweden, maintains a moving 5-year plan of expenditure and development, plus a longer term plan that is more general in nature. The latter, recently updated to cover the whole of the 1980s, covers such items as numbers of hospital beds, changing emphases in care, manpower needs and creation of new hospitals and community clinics. The 5-year plan must accord with the longer plan, and is the main vehicle for implementation of the policies and ideas of that farther-reaching document.

The revised 5-year plan that covers 1976-1980 was approved progressively during late 1975 and early 1976. One section of this, occupying 70 pages, related to E.D.P. developments. Prepared by the finance directorate in conjunction with appropriate staffs, but receiving the imprint of authority through Council approval, this document gives a picture of the present status and the intended development of each computer application, along with financial estimates.

In discussing the medical applications, the primary point made is that the main part of resource consumption is due to medical decisions, so it is logical to seek, through development of the information system, a better basis for such decisions. Thereby will the patient receive better care, while an ancillary goal is to increase the effectiveness of clinic staffs and facilities, including by lightening the administrative load. The emphasis is thus on less tangible benefits, but, by illustrating how the System has allowed earlier service to waiting patients for the major ophthalmic clinic and mitigated what had been seen as a chronic under-provision of facilities, the financial gain can be appreciated if not quantified. The savings derived through removal of clinical work from nursing areas can generally be quantified, but usually amount to fragmentary savings that are not directly realizable. They are typically translated into improved care. Realizable savings are regarded as only those covering whole staff positions or external expenditures.

Only the inpatient application, inclusive of waiting list and inpatient sub-system, is estimated as having major tangible benefits at present. However, inclusive of the non-realizable benefits, the gain is less than half the assessed cost of 5 million crowns per annum, though this is foreseen as improving significantly over the coming years. The prime realizable benefits, relative to the preceding batch system, arise from the avoidance of key-punching (36 employees) and of separate error checking (3 employees), the abandonment of admission/discharge forms (100 000 crowns p.a.) and the automatic production of daily census and other reports (6 employees), plus the saving of batch computer time. The release of nursing area staffs from manual preparation of patient directory and census data is estimated to save some 20 minutes per day per nursing station, which, together with concomitant savings in central offices, will be worth 1.7 million crowns as the older procedures are phased out by 1977. Minor development to cover certain accounting data will add 10% to this figure, which is classed as non-realizable. The costs - predominantly central computing but including additional user costs as well as the terminals - are seen as rising for a time then declining as greater utilization of equipment lowers the proportional charges. Table 14-2 gives the estimated figures, plus an interpretation of the net additional cost per admission and per ward-day. These are seen as rising then falling also, but with figures generally close to 10 crowns ($2.50) and 0.35 crowns ($0.10) respectively, after allowing for non-realizable benefits. The gross cost

	1975	1976	1977	1978	1979	1980
NEW COSTS						
USER PERSONNEL	700	790	750	690	690	690
DATACENTRAL	3 361	3 738	3 635	3 510	3 220	3 040
TERMINALS	1 050	1 540	1 320	1 320	1 320	1 320
TOTAL	5 111	6 068	5 705	5 520	5 230	5 050
AVOIDED COSTS						
USER PERSONNEL	300	450	600	600	600	600
FORMS	50	80	125	125	125	125
COMPUTING	1 000	1 800	1 800	1 800	1 800	1 800
TOTAL	1 350	2 330	2 525	2 525	2 525	2 525
NON-REALIZABLE	800	1 300	1 860	1 860	1 860	1 860
TOTAL	2 150	3 630	4 385	4 385	4 385	4 385
NET COST						
TOTAL	2 961	2 438	1 320	1 135	845	665
PER 1000 CASES	13.2	13.3	11.0	10.2	9.0	8.4
PER 1000 BED-DAYS	0.46	0.47	0.39	0.36	0.32	0.30
VOLUME						
1000 CASES	282	282	288	294	300	300
1000 BED-DAYS	8 000	8 000	8 100	8 300	8 500	8 500

TABLE 14-2 BUDGET FOR INPATIENT APPLICATION (EXPRESSED IN THOUSANDS OF CROWNS)

would be about five times these figures.

Current network expenditures for all applications are included in Table 14-3, which provides a break-up of the 1975 costs for medical E.D.P. The figure for the inpatient application differs from that of Table 14-2 because of one being an estimate made prior to the year-end. This further table, like Table 14-1, omits any expenditures incurred outside Datacentral and the terminal network, so does not cover all additional costs.

Besides the direct cost of the various application sub-systems, it should be noted there is a considerable cost for updating the H.R., and a still greater cost for the miscellaneous real-time enquiries thereto, and

	DATACENTRAL						
	REAL-TIME PROCESSES	BATCH PROCESSES	DEVICE STORAGE	DATA INPUT	DEVELOP -MENT	TOTAL	TERMINALS
INPATIENT	436	1 677	163	286	556	3 118	1 050
BOOKING	369	549	117	3	174	1 212	96
OUTPATIENT	204	69	47	2	23	345	600
CHEM LAB	1 309	749	232	3	280	2 573	90
X-RAY		286		451	78	815	
H.R. UPDATING		177		1	109	287	
H.R. ENQUIRIES	417				23	440	700
GENERAL REAL-TIME	3	132	224	5	249	613	92
GENERAL BATCH							
TOTAL	2 738	4 233	783	862	1 882	13 126	2 628

<u>TABLE</u> 14-3 BREAK-UP OF 1975 MEDICAL E.D.P. EXPENDITURES.
(EXPRESSED IN THOUSANDS OF CROWNS.)

yet more for the general real-time routines, from dialog analysis to file compression. Hence the cost of the composite inpatient application would be significantly higher than previously stated should the other applications be discontinued, and in any case should be inflated by about 10% to cover these overheads.

Of the other applications, only the chemical laboratory sub-system is seen as having tangible benefits, amounting to a realizable 60 000 crowns in 1975 through automatic preparation of laboratory lists and reports, plus an unrealizable 600 000 crowns from automatic handling of requisitions and outgoing reports. However, these barely offset other additional costs at the time. The current net cost of 2.6 million crowns represents about 1.7 crowns per analysis. Tables 14-4 & 14-5 give the budget for outpatient and, laboratory applications respectively, with both showing massive increases in expenditure as N-development allow wider implementation.

The booking sub-system, inclusive of extra costs in the Health Department, currently costs about 1.4 million crowns p.a., or about 17 crowns per booking. Some decline, to about 12 crowns per booking, is foreseen within the extant development.

<u>Plans for further development</u>

Major revision of the booking, outpatient and chemical laboratory sub-systems is planned before these are expanded further in coverage.

The greatest drawback with the extant booking sub-system is over-sophistication. Designed to have one dialog cover up to nine appointments with in-built time-spacing and sequencing, the programs offered facilities beyond what the user in practice wanted - at the price of complication to the user and both program space and execution time within the computer. While the display aspect can be simplified, the programs must be revised substantially to bring their execution costs down to a satisfactory level. Simultaneously with this reduction in sophistication, various additional features need to be added to enhance the value of the booking sub-system, including procedures that would automatically fill most vacancies with patients from the waiting list, once a certain period had elapsed, while leaving a residue for urgent cases. More connection is required between these two sub-systems for daily planning purposes, while various analysis and statistical routines are needed in the booking sub-system to assist monthly and longer-term planning. A closer coupling with the laboratory sub-system is also required. No budget is currently assigned to re-development of the booking sub-system, for which current costs are expressly identified as experimental.

The outpatient sub-system, although taking only a modest proportion of current E.D.P. expenditures, is very expensive relative to its coverage. The pilot implementation at Huddinge covers barely 100 000 visits per year, or 2% of the County total. The provision of computer terminals is certainly lavish, but even the cost at Datacentral alone would make multiplication by 50 unacceptable. As discussed below, computer capacity alone would inhibit such escalation, while the widespread of sources for outpatient data, extending to local clinics and doctors offices, makes collection difficult. Extended implementation is thus seen as requiring both optical reading of documents and improved computer processes as means of economising. On the other hand, extension of the programs to cover accounting aspects, plus closer integration with other sub-systems, are seen as imperative for economic acceptability.

Development and full implementation of such a revised sub-system for outpatients is included in the current 5-year plan, and initial development is underway. As is shown in Table 14-4, this will bring a vast increase in the related operational costs at Datacentral, and demand considerable expenses for training and other new staff in the field. Indeed, with this horizon, the sub-system will cause an increase in staff. The net cost is estimated as being close to 1 crown per outpatient visit, and is justified by the abilities thereby created for analysis of care, on individual and statistical bases.

	1975	1976	1977	1978	1979	1980
NEW COSTS						
FORMS	0	25	100	150	200	250
USER STAFF	60	60	128	180	240	240
ACCTG. STAFF			100	150	200	250
DEV. STAFF	70	200	200	150	150	70
DATACENTRAL	630	908	1 000	2 000	3 000	4 000
TERMINALS	600	560	440	550	660	770
TOTAL	1 360	1 753	1 960	3 180	4 450	5 580
AVOIDED COSTS						
MISSED INCOME			50	75	100	125
PERSONNEL			50	100	150	200
TOTAL	0	0	100	175	250	325
NET COST						
TOTAL	1 360	1 753	1 860	3 005	4 200	5 255
PER 1000 VISITS	13.2	14.8	15.5	1.5	1.2	1.0
VOLUME						
1000 VISITS	104	119	119	1 940	3 560	5 200

TABLE 14-4 BUDGET FOR OUTPATIENT SUB-SYSTEM.
(EXPRESSED IN THOUSANDS OF CROWNS.)

Major revision of the chemical laboratory sub-system hinges on the introduction of mini-computers for collection and primary processing of data within the major laboratory complexes, inclusive of on-line coupling to automatic laboratory instruments. As the budget in Table 14-5 shows, this is expected to increase the gross annual cost by about 70% over the five years, while increasing the coverage of the sub-system from about 1.5 million tests per annum to the envisaged County total of 10 million per annum in 1980. The high degree of automatic data processing and transmission that will be reached by the revised sub-system is estimated to yield tangible benefits that will be close to the gross cost, reducing post-analysis net cost from the present 1.73 crowns to 0.008 crowns. For this minor unit expense both quality and responsiveness should be improved significantly in relation to laboratory reports.

1975	1976		1977	1978	1979	1980
NEW COSTS						
USER STAFF	365	70	210	210	210	210
DEV. STAFF	120	120	120	120	40	40
DATACENTRAL	2 685	2 504	2 750	3 454	3 835	3 830
TERMINALS	90	84	88	110	154	154
MINI COMPS	0	400	550	1 000	1 000	1 000
TOTAL	3 260	3 178	3 718	4 894	5 239	5 234
AVOIDED COSTS						
REALIZABLE	60	120	130	215	370	410
NON-REALIZABLE	600	1 500	1 500	2 750	4 000	4 000
TOTAL	660	1 620	1 630	2 965	4 370	4 410
NET COSTS						
TOTAL	2 600	1 558	2 088	1 929	869	824
PER 1000 ANALYSES	1.733	.600	.774	.386	.097	.080
VOLUME						
1000 ANALYSES	1 500	2 600	2 700	5 000	9 000	10 000

TABLE 14-5 BUDGET FOR CHEMICAL LABORATORY SUB-SYSTEM. (EXPRESSED IN THOUSANDS OF CROWNS.)

Beyond the five identified real-time sub-systems, the x-ray application, although reliant on batch updating, has a major real-time component through the on-line reference to the investigational reports in the H.R. It is planned that the updating also be done via terminals as a real-time process, and an experimental operation was instituted in 1975. Conversion to real-time of the data input will require both terminals and associated operators in considerable numbers - estimated as costing 0.5 million crowns and 0.253 million crowns respectively for the full volume of a million investigations per year; however, central computing and keypunching costs are seen as comparably reduced. After the initial development years, it is estimated that this particular development will be profitable, relative to the current batch-update process. The cost of data processing per investigation is estimated to fall from the current 1.50 crowns to nil. In addition, the application will make the current status available to the H.R. enquiry, helping to obviate unnecessary filming; it will also enhance monitoring of exposure of patients to x-rays.

In all these applications, progressive expansion of coverage means closer approximation to the target of comprehensive machine-analyzable records of health care utilization, with concomitant advantages to both the provision of facilities and the planning of care protocols. As the knowledge on treatments accumulates, formal therapeutic plans are being assembled both as representative measuring bases for scheduling and as starting bases for ordering individual therapy regimes.

APPENDIX A

BACKGROUND DATA CONCERNING STOCKHOLM COUNTY

SHORT-TERM SOMATIC CARE	7 789
SHORT-TERM PSYCHIATRIC CARE	5 061
LONG-TERM CARE	9 245
PRIVATE NURSING HOMES	1 944
NURSING HOMES FOR THE ELDERLY	788
PRIVATE PSYCHIATRIC NURSING HOMES	528
CONVALESCENT HOMES	154
PRIVATE CONVALESCENT HOMES	217
TOTAL	25 726

TABLE A-1 NUMBERS OF BEDS IN STOCKHOLM COUNTY, 1976

(EXCEPT WHERE DENOTED AS "PRIVATE", ALL BEDS ARE OPERATED BY THE COUNTY)
OF THE 7 789 SHORT-TERM SOMATIC CARE BEDS, APPROXIMATELY 44% ARE FOR MEDICINE, 50% FOR SURGERY AND 6% FOR PAEDIATRICS; GYNAECOLOGY AND OPHTHALMOLOGY ARE CLASSIFIED AS SUB-SPECIALTIES OF SURGERY.

	SW. CR.
MEDICAL SERVICES	
DENTAL SERVICES	175 000
WELFARE OF MENTALLY RETARDED	300 000
GENERAL REHABILITATION	195 000
GENERAL SOPCIAL WELFARE	91 000
TRAFFIC MANAGEMENT	612 000
ADULT AND SPECIAL EDUCATION	119 000
TOTAL	4 820 000

TABLE A-2 EXPENSE BUDGET FOR STOCKHOLM COUNTY 1976

ABOUT 53% OF ALL EXPENSES RELATE TO SALARIES, 15% TO CONTRACTED SERVICES AND 9% TO CAPITAL PURCHASES.
STATE GRANTS AND MINOR CONTRIBUTIONS FROM SERVICED MUNICIPALITIES PROVIDE 42% OF INCOME, AND FEES FOR MEDICAL SERVICES 37%.

PERSONNEL POSITIONS

PHYSICIANS	1 435	
GENERAL NURSES	4 582	
PSYCHIATRIC NURSES	2 070	
NURSING AUXILIARIES	8 845	
DOMESTIC STAFF	2 631	
OFFICE STAFF*	2 335	
OTHER	4 599	
TOTAL		27 294

PATIENTS

REGISTERED POPULATION	1 500 000
ADMISSIONS	272 070
BED DAYS	8 140 640
OUTPATIENT VISITS	4 816 515

COSTS PER PATIENT BED-DAY

NEPHROLOGY	1 350 SW.CR.
NEUROSURGERY	860 SW.CR.
OTORHINOLARYNGOLOGY	610 SW.CR.
GENERAL SURGERY	540 SW.CR.
MEDICINE	430 SW.CR.
LONG-TERM HOSPITAL	235 SW.CR.

TABLE A-3 MISCELLANEOUS HEALTH-CARE STATISTICS FOR STOCKHOLM COUNTY, 1976.

*AS MENTIONED IN THE TEXT, MANY OFFICE SERVICES ARE PROVIDED BY OTHER ARMS OF THE COUNTY FOR HEALTH CARE ALONG WITH OTHER ACTIVITIES

APPENDIX B

CODES

ANEC ANAESTHESIA CODE

CIV (CIVIL STATUS) IS A 1-DIGIT CODE WITH THE FOLLOWING VALUES

VALUE	MEANING
1	UNMARRIED ADULT
2	MARRIED MAN
3	SEPARATED WIFE
4	DIVORCED
5	WIDOWED
6	DECEASED
7	WIFE
8	CHILD UNDER 18 YEARS
9	FOSTER CHILD UNDER 18 YEARS

DRUGC (DRUG CODE) IS AN 8- CHARACTER CODE INVOLVING ONE SPACE CHARACTER, BUT USUALLY BEING ONE CHARACTER SHORT OF MAXIMAL. PRECEDING THE SPACE IS A DRUG-GROUP IDENTIFIER, BEING A NUMBER IN THE RANGE 1, 2,... 13, PLUS ONE LETTER. FOLLOWING THE SPACE IS A 4-DIGIT SERIAL NUMBER WITHIN THE GROUP. EXAMPLES OF THE GROUP IDENTIFIER, EXAMPLES OF CODES THEREIN, ARE

2F	DIEURETICS AND POTASSIUM
2F	0550 FURO-SEMID
7A	SULFA DRUGS
7A	0517 SULFAFUROZOLE
7B	ANTIBIOTICS
7B	2505 STREPTOMYCIN
7C	DRUGS AGAINST SPECIAL INFECTIONS
7C	4005 NITROFURATOIN
10H	THYROID HORMONES AND ANTI-THYROID SUBSTANCES
10H	0505 LEVOTYROXIN

THE CODE IS USUALLY ENTERED IN TERMINALS WITHOUT THE EMBEDDED SPACE, I.E. AS A 6- OR 7- CHARACTER ENTRY, LEFT JUSTIFIED.

DEPT (DEPARTMENT) HAS BEEN USED, RELATIVE TO THE INTERNAL ORGANIZATION OF HOSPITALS ETC., TO COVER MEDICAL DEPARTMENTS AND WHAT ARE OFTEN, IN N. AMERICA, DIVISIONS OF SUCH DEPARTMENTS. A 3-DIGIT CODE IS USED, WITH COMMON INFERENCE FOR ANY VALUE ACROSS ALL INSTITUTIONS - THOUGH WITH VALUES FREQUENTLY SET FOR ONE PARTICULAR INSTITUTION. DIFFERENT VALUES CAN HAVE THE SAME NAME, IF TWO OR MORE SIMILAR UNITS NEED TO BE IDENTIFIED.
EXAMPLES

VALUE	UNIT
141	ALLERGIES
151	DIALYSIS
161	ENDOCRINOLOGY
171	INDUSTRIAL MEDICINE
301	(GENERAL) SURGERY
302	(GENERAL) SURGERY
311	ORTHOPAEDICS
411	ANAESTHESIA
421	SPECIAL ANAESTHESIA
441	OBSTETRICAL DELIVERIES
711	PATHOLOGY
715	CYTOLOGY
901 THRU 905	PSYCHIATRY

EACH SUCH UNIT HAS ALSO A 2- OR 3-LETTER SHORT NAME E.G. DIA = DIALYSIS, ORT = ORTHOPAEDICS, PAT = PATHOLOGY.

E, E1, ETC SEE EXAM

EXAM IS A 4-DIGIT CODE IDENTIFYING THE VARIOUS INVESTIGATORY, DIAGNOSTIC AND THERAPEUTIC PROCEDURES AVAILABLE TO PATIENTS, RANGING FROM THE SPECIFICITY - OF A PARTICULAR TEST TO THE BROADNESS OF "RETURN VISIT" TO A PARTICULAR DEPARTMENT. THE CODE IS CURRENTLY APPLIED INDEPENDENTLY WITHIN EACH PARTICIPATING INSTITUTION, ALTHOUGH THE MODEST NUMBERS OF VALUES USED HAVE ALLOWED DISJOINT SUB-RANGES TO BE ASSIGNED EACH HOSPITAL. EXAMPLES

WITHIN ONE HOSPITAL

0130 MYELOGRAM
0203 BRONCHOGRAM
0220 ANGIOGRAM
0450 CHOLECYSTOGRAM
0642 X-RAY OF KNEE AND LOWER LEG

WITHIN ANOTHER HOSPITAL
1010 NEW VISIT TO MEDICINE DEPT.
1011 RETURN VISIT TO MEDICINE DEPT.
1020 NEW VISIT TO MEDICINE DEPT. (I.E. WITH DIFFERENT TIME OR OTHER PARAMETERS)
1085 RETURN VISIT AFTER INPATIENT STAY
9020 RETURN VISIT TO DR. E.

INSTN (INSTITUTION) IS A 5-DIGIT CODE IDENTIFYING THE INDIVIDUAL HOSPITALS, NEIGHBORHOOD CLINICS, ETC., THAT PROVIDE THE HEALTH SERVICES. THE CODE WAS ESTABLISHED WITH AN INTENTION OF HAVING IN-BUILT SIGNIFICANCE. HOWEVER, ALTHOUGH SOME SUCH CONSTRUCTION OCCURS, ALL CURRENT VALUES ARE IN THE RANGE 10001 THRU 11999. EXAMPLES

VALUE	INSTITUTION
11001	KAROLINSKA
11002	HUDDINGE
11010	DANDERYD

EACH INSTITUTION ALSO HAS A 2-, 3- OR 4-LETTER SHORT NAME EG. KS, HS AND DS, WHERE THE 'S' STANDS FOR THE SWEDISH SJUKHUSET (=HOSPITAL).

OPNC OPERATION CODE

PERSON-NUMB. THE STANDARD SWEDISH PERSONAL IDENTIFICATION NUMBER ('PERSONNUMMER'), OF THE FORM
YYMMDD@RRSC

WHERE YYMMDD IS YEAR-MONTH-DAY OF BIRTH
@ = + FOR BIRTHS BEFORE 1900, - FOR OTHERS
RR = REGION OF REGISTRATION
S = SEQUENCE NUMBER: EVEN FOR FEMALES, ODD FOR MALES
C = MODULO-10 CHECK DIGIT

PNR SEE PERSON-NUMB

PNR/RNR SEE PNR AND RNR

PRTY (PRIORITY) A 1- OR 2-LETTER CODE BASED ON STANDARDS SET BY THE SOCIAL WELFARE AUTHORITY, BEING

VALUE	MEANING
FF	PATIENT SHOULD HAVE SERVICE WITHIN 6 DAYS
F	PATIENT SHOULD HAVE SERVICE WITHIN 6 WEEKS
N	PATIENT CAN WAIT MORE THAN 6 WEEKS
I	PATIENT CAN WAIT INDEFINITELY - I.E. ULTRA-LOW PRIORITY, EQUIVALENT TO "UNNECESSARY" AS APPLIED TO RELATED DEMAND.

THE VALUE P IS ALSO USED IN THE SAME FIELD TO INDICATE THAT A BOOKING HAS BEEN MADE.

R, R1, ETC., SEE RESOURCE

RESOURCE IS A 4-DIGIT CODE IDENTIFYING THE EXPLICIT RESOURCES ABLE TO PROVIDE THE INVESTIGATORY DIAGNOSTIC AND THEREAPEUTIC SERVICES. THE DEFINITION OF THE CODE VALUES ARE ESSENTIALLY RELATIVE TO INSTITUTION - I.E. A VALUE CAN HAVE DIFFERENT MEANINGS IN DIFFERENT HOSPITALS. THE FORM OF IDENTIFIED RESOURCE CAN VARY EVEN WITHIN A DEPARTMENT, BEING A ROOM FOR SOME THINGS, A MACHINE FOR OTHERS, A SPECIFIC PERSON FOR OTHERS. EXAMPLES

1020 MEDICINE DEPT. - DR ERIK O
1021 MEDICINE DEPT. - DR JOHN M

7309 X-RAY, DIGESTIVE TRACT, UNIT 1
7310 X-RAY, DIGESTIVE TRACT, UNIT 2

7340 X-RAY, THORAX

7380 X-RAY, SPECIAL PROCEDURES, ROOM 1
7381 X-RAY, SPECIAL PROCEDURES, ROOM 2

EACH RESOURCE IS ALSO ACCORDED A SHORT NAME, LIMIT 9 CHARACTERS

RESV-NUMBER IS THE SUBSTITUTE NUMBER FOR VISITORS, NEWBORNS AND OTHERS NOT REGISTERED IN THE SYSTEM WITH A PERSON-NUMB. THIS SUBSTITUTE NUMBER EMBEDS THE INSTITUTION REQUIRING IT -HENCE, IN FACT, A PATIENT MAY HAVE MORE THAN ONE SUCH NUMBER.

RNR SEE RESV-NUMBER

APPENDIX C

DATA TERMINAL CHARACTERISTICS

DATA ENTRY KEYS

THE DATA ENTRY KEYS ARE USED FOR INPUT OF ALPHABETIC CHARACTERS, NUMERIC CHARACTERS AND SPECIAL SIGNS. THE FUNCTIONS ARE SUMMARIZED IN THE FOLLOWING TABLE.

KEY	NO SHIFT	SHIFT
SHIFT		ENABLES SELECTION OF SPECIAL CHARACTERS ON UPPER HALF OF KEYS OR PROVIDES SHIFT FUNCTIONS FOR EDIT AND PROGRAM KEYS.
SINGLE CHARACTER	CAUSES THE CHARACTER TO BE DISPLAYED IN THE CURSOR POSITION AND MOVES CURSOR TO THE NEXT CHARACTER POSITION.	SAME
DOUBLE CHARACTER KEYS	CAUSES CHARACTER ON LOWER HALF OF KEY TO BE DISPLAYED IN THE CURSOR POSITION AND MOVES CURSOR TO THE NEXT CHARACTER POSITION	CAUSES CHARACTER ON UPPER HALF OF KEY TO BE DISPLAYED IN THE CURSOR POSITION AND MOVES CURSOR TO THE NEXT CHARACTER POSITION
SPACE	ADVANCES THE CURSOR ONE CHARACTER POSITION TO THE RIGHT AND LEAVES A BLANK SPACE BETWEEN THE LAST CHARACTER AND THE CURSOR. IF CURSOR IS POSITIONED ON AN ALREADY CREATED CHARACTER, THE CHARACTER IS LOST.	SAME
UNDERLINE KEY	CAUSES THE CHARACTER ZERO TO BE DISPLAYED IN THE CURSOR POSITION AND MOVES CURSOR TO THE NEXT CHARACTER POSITION	GIVES UNDERLINING OR FLASHING OF THE SUCCEEDING CHARACTERS UNTIL A SPACE OR END OF LINE APPEARS. CURSOR MOVES TO THE NEXT CHARACTER POSITION

EDIT KEYS

THE FUNCTION OF THE EDIT KEYS ARE SUMMARIZED IN THE FOLLOWING TABLE:

KEY	NO SHIFT	SHIFT
START	PUTS START OF MESSAGE CHARACTER IN CURSOR POSITION. CURSOR MOVES TO NEXT CHARACTER POSITION	SAME
NEW LINE	MOVES THE CURSOR TO THE FIRST POSITION OF THE NEXT LINE. IF ALREADY ON LINE 16 OF THE SCREEN, THE CURSOR WRAPS AROUND TO THE FIRST POSITION ON THE FIRST LINE, AND AN AUDIBLE ALARM SIGNAL IS GIVEN. THE CHARACTER IN THE ORIGINAL POSITION IS NOT AFFECTED	MOVES THE CURSOR TO THE FIRST CHARACTER POSITION ON THE SAME LINE
CURSOR CONTROL	MOVES CURSOR ONE CHARACTER POSITION IN THE DIRECTION INDICATED BY THE ARROW ON THE KEY. AN AUTOMATIC CURSOR MOVEMENT STARTS AFTER 0.5 SECONDS IF THE KEY IS KEPT DEPRESSED	SAME
HOME/CLEAR	MOVES THE CURSOR TO THE FIRST POSITION ON THE FIRST LINE	ERASES ALL TEXT ON THE SCREEN AND MOVES THE CURSOR TO THE FIRST POSITION ON THE FIRST LINE

KEY	NO SHIFT	SHIFT
INSERT CHARACTER/ ERASE LINE	MOVES THE TEXT-LINE TO THE RIGHT OF AND INCLUDING THE CURSOR POSITION ONE CHARACTER POSITION TO THE RIGHT. THE LAST CHARACTER ON THE LINE IS LOST	ERASES ALL TEXT TO THE RIGHT OF AND INCLUDING THE CURSOR POSITION TO THE LAST POSITION OF THE LINE
DELETE CHARACTER/ ERASE SCREEN	MOVES THE TEXT-LINE TO THE RIGHT OF THE CURSOR ONE CHARACTER POSITION TO THE LEFT. THE CHARACTER OCCUPYING THE CURSOR POSITION IS DELETED	ERASES ALL TEXT TO THE RIGHT OF AND INCLUDING THE CURSOR POSITION TO THE LAST POSITION ON THE SCREEN'
LINE INSERT/ LINE DELETE	MOVES THE LINE AT THE CURSOR POSITION AND ALL FOLLOWING LINES DOWN ONE LINE, RESULTING IN A BLANK LINE AT THE CURSOR POSITION AND LOSS OF LINE 16	DELETES THE LINE AT THE CURSOR POSITION AND MOVES THE LINES BELOW UP ONE LINE CAUSING A BLANK LINE 16
TABULATION	MOVES THE CURSOR TO THE FIRST/ SECOND POSITION TO THE RIGHT OF THE NEXT FORMAT STOP OR TAB SET CHARACTER. IF THERE IS NO FORMAT STOP OR TAB SET CHARACTER ON THE SCREEN, THE CURSOR WILL NOT MOVE	SAME
REPEAT	THE LAST SELECTED CHARACTER OR FUNCTION IS AUTOMATICALLY REPEATED AT A CONSTANT RATE OF TEN CHARACTERS PER SECOND. THE CHARACTER KEY SHALL NOT BE DEPRESSED SIMULTANEOUSLY WITH THE REPEAT KEY.	SAME

2613 2618

FUNCTION KEYS

THE FUNCTION KEYS OPERATE INDEPENDENTLY OF THE SHIFT KEY POSITION. THE KEYS ARE AS FOLLOWS

RESET KEY	WHEN THE KEY IS DEPRESSED THE DISPLAY SET WILL BE RESET TO RECEIVING MODE. THE USE OF THE RESET KEY WILL E.G. INHIBIT INITIATED BUT NOT EXECUTED DATA TRANSMISSION AND PRINTOUT. THE KEYBOARD WILL UNLOCK WHEN THIS KEY IS DEPRESSED EXCEPT DURING DATA TRANSMISSION.
CLEAR KEY	ERASES ALL TEXT (INCLUDING PROTECTED FIELDS) FROM AND INCLUDING THE CURSOR POSITION TO THE END OF THE SCREEN INCLUSIVE THE PROGRAM LINE (LINE 17).
USM KEY	WHEN THE COMPUTER HAS AN UNSOLICITED MESSAGE TO SEND TO THE DISPLAY SET THE LAMP IN THIS KEY STARTS FLASHING. DEPRESSING THE KEY TURNS OFF THE LAMP AND THE DISPLAY SET IS READY TO RECEIVE THE MESSAGE.

PRINTOUT KEY — THIS KEY IS USED TO INITIATE PRINTOUT OF DATA BETWEEN THE LAST START OF MESSAGE CHARACTER AND THE CURSOR. IF NO START OF MESSAGE CHARACTER EXCISTS BEFORE THE CURSOR, THE PRINTOUT STARTS FROM THE FIRST POSITION ON THE FIRST LINE.

WHEN THE PRINT KEY IS DEPRESSED, THE KEYBOARD IS LOCKED DURING THE PRINTOUT. IF THE PRINTER IS OCCUPIED WITH PRINTOUTS ORDERED FROM OTHER DISPLAY SETS CONNECTED TO THE SAME DISPLAY CONTROLLER, OR BY THE COMPUTER, THE KEYBOARD WILL BE LOCKED DURING THESE PRINTOUTS. THE KEYBOARD CAN BE UNLOCKED BY DEPRESSING THE RESET KEY IF AN OPERATOR DOES NOT WANT TO WAIT FOR THE PRINTER READY STATUS.

PRINT-REQUEST KEY — THIS KEY IS USED TO INITIATE A PRINTOUT VIA THE COMMUNICATION COMPUTER. WHEN THE KEY IS DEPRESSED, DATA FROM THE LAST START OF MESSAGE TO END OF TEXT, OR BETWEEN THE FIRST SCREEN POSITION AND END OF TEXT CHARACTER IS TRANSMITTED TO THE COMPUTER.

SEND KEY — WHEN THIS KEY IS PRESSED THE END OF TEXT CHARACTER IS ENTERED IN THE CURSOR POSITION AND THE CURSOR STOPS FLASHING. DATA INCLUDING THE LAST START OF MESSAGE TO END OF TEXT CHARACTER, OR IF THERE IS NO START OF MESSAGE CHARACTER, DATA FROM THE FIRST SCREEN POSITION TO END OF TEXT CHARACTER, IS TRANSMITTED TO THE COMPUTER.

THE KEYBOARD IS LOCKED DURING THE TRANSMISSION AND THE CURSOR IS MOVED ALONG THE MESSAGE TO BE TRANSMITTED. ON COMPLETION OF TRANSMISSION THE CURSOR OCCUPIES THE POSITION OF THE END OF TEXT CHARACTER.

THE END OF TEXT CHARACTER IS ERASED AFTER A COMPLETE TRANSMISSION.

PROGRAM KEYS

THE UPPER ROW OF THE KEYBOARD COMPRISES FIVE PROGRAM KEYS P1-P5. WHEN A PROGRAM KEY IS DEPRESSED, A SPECIAL CODE SEQUENCE CONSISTING OF A HEADER AND FOUR CHARACTERS IS TRANSMITTED TO THE COMPUTER. THE FIVE PROGRAM KEYS CAN GENERATE TEN PROGRAM CODE SEQUENCES BY USING THE SHIFT KEY.

ON THE PROGRAM LINE (LINE 17), WHICH CAN BE ADDRESSED ONLY FROM THE COMPUTER, THE OPERATOR CAN BE INFORMED OF THE PROGRAM KEYS FUNCTION IN THE RUNNING PROGRAM.